# Current Developments
# in Psychopharmacology

# Current Developments in Psychopharmacology

## Volume 6

**EDITORS**

**Walter B. Essman**
Departments of Psychology & Biochemistry
Queens College of the City University of New York,
Flushing, N.Y.

**L. Valzelli**
Section of Neuropsychopharmacology
Mario Negri Institute for Pharmacological Research
Milan, Italy

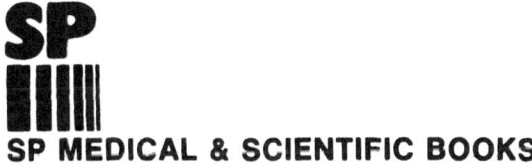

**SP MEDICAL & SCIENTIFIC BOOKS**
New York

Spectrum Publications, Inc.
175-20 Wexford Terrace, Jamaica, New York 11432

ISBN-13: 978-94-011-8125-9      e-ISBN-13: 978-94-011-8123-5
DOI: 10.1007/978-94-011-8123-5

*Library of Congress Catalogue Card Number: 75-502*

# CURRENT DEVELOPMENTS IN PSYCHOPHARMACOLOGY

**Volume 1**
Dopamine Receptors and Their Role in Brain Function *(Barnett)*; Brain Serotonergic and Catecholamine Systems: Facts and Hypothesis *(Kostowski)*; Hippocampal and Autonomic Pharmacology in Performance and Learning *(Izquierdo)*; Pharmacological and Neurochemical Approaches to Memory Trace Retrieval *(Ilyutchenok)*; Cerebral Biochemical and Pharmacological Changes in Differentially Housed Mice *(DeFeudis)*; Rubidium in Psychiatry and Medicine: An Overview *(Meltzer* and *Fieve)*; Clinical Psychopharmacology of the Affective Disorders *(Abrams)*; Drug Effects in the Assessment of Affective States in Man *(Gottschalk)*; Cerebral Electrometry in Phase-1 Assessment of Psychoactive Drugs *(Fink)*; Subject Index; Author Index

**Volume 2**
Studies of Central Cholinergic Neurons *(Kuhar, Simon* and *Rommelspacher)*; Flurothyl–Pharmacology of Seizures in Animals and Man *(Adler)*; The Clinical Use of Flurothyl *(Small* and *Small)*; The Action of Central Nervous System Stimulant Drugs: A General Theory Concerning Amphetamine Effects *(Lyon* and *Robbins)*; Advances in the Search for Improved Neuroleptic Drugs *(Janssen* and *Van Bever)*; Sensory Psychopharmacology *(Robinson* and *Sabat)*; Mania, Depression, and Brain Dopamine *(Randrup, Munkvad, Fog, Gerlach, Molander, Kjellberg* and *Scheel-Krüger)*

**Volume 3**
Amnesia and the Biology of Memory *(Squire)*; Cycloheximide: Mechanisms of its Amnesic Effect *(Nakajima)*; Piracetam: Nootropic Pharmacology of Neurointegrative Activity *(Giurgea)*; Dopaminergic Drug Effects upon Serotoninergic Neurons *(Maj)*; Neurotransmitter Regulation of Pituitary Secretion *(Rose* and *Ganong)*; Aminergic Factors in Mental Illness *(Berger)*; Mechanisms of Lithium Toxicity Development in Rats *(Thomsen, Olesen* and *Jensen)*; Drug Therapy in Depressive States: Factors in Suicide Prevention *(Poeldinger)*; Drug Induced Aggression *(Gianutsos* and *Lal)*

**Volume 4**
Opiate Receptors in the Central Nervous System *(Simon)*; Pharmacological and Biochemical Studies with β-Carboline Analogs *(Ho)*; Recent Advances in Genetics and Psychopharmacology *(Mendlewicz)*; Psychopharmacology of Aging: Current Trends *(Sathananthan, Gershon,* and *Ferris)*; Catecholamines and Behavior *(Engel* and *Carlsson)*; Neuropharmacology of Hyperkinesis *(Silbergeld)*; Long Term Treatment with Neuroleptics in Psychiatry *(Shepherd* and *Watt)*; Precipitated Morphine Withdrawal in Rats as a Tool in Opiate Research *(Bläsig* and *Herz)*; Tricyclic Antidepressants: A Review of Their Toxicology *(Fiori)*

**Volume 5**

The Pharmacology of Isolation-Induced Aggressive Behavior in Mice *(Malick)*; Neurochemical Issues in Animal and Human Behavior *(Valzelli)*; Circadian Rhythms in Manic-Melancholic Disorders *(Mellerup and Rafaelsen)*; Pituitary Hormones and Amnesia *(Rigter and Riezen)*; The Effects of D-Amphetamine on Dopaminergic Regulated Mechanism of Physiological and Behavioral Thermoregulation *(Yehuda)*; Metabolism and Functions of Histamine in the Brain *(Schwartz, Barbin, Baudry, Gargarg, Martres, Pollard, and Verdiere)*; Psychobiological Interactions and Schizophrenia *(Shore)*; Serotonin and Affective Disorders *(Burns and Mendels)*; Clinical Language and Communication as a Tool of Psychopharmacological Research *(Andreoli and Maffei)*; Sex Steroid Control of Intermale Fighting in Mice *(Brain and Bowden)*

# Preface

The areas of experimental and clinical psychopharmacology have continued to grow in terms of the numbers of studies appearing in the literature as well as the activity generated by other disciplines that has influenced the output of behavioral pharmacology research. Psychoactive drugs have been considered for their comparative effects upon selected behaviors or for their effect upon diverse behaviors. Behavioral circumstances certainly influence not only the metabolism and action of psychotropic drugs behaviorally, but also the disposition of these agents and/or their metabolites in regions of the central nervous system. There can hardly be a psychopharmacology without a neuropharmacology, and the latter would seem to depend upon a neurochemistry. There would appear to be variables that exert potent influences upon the disposition and action of psychotropic drugs, that also relate quite directly to their effects upon behavior; these include drug interactions, nutritional status, environmental effects such as temperature, photic and tactile stimulation, and stress, and the basal status upon which such drug treatment is superimposed.

In this volume of *Current Developments in Psychopharmacology*, which will be the last to appear in this format, we have sought to focus upon a series of current topical reviews that highlight representative areas of experimental and clinical research activity in psychopharmacology. In the first chapter, Dr. Lagerspetz reviews a frequently neglected aspect of psychopharmacological research—the actions of psychoactive agents upon the nervous system and behavior of non-mammalian species. Such comparative psychopharmacology presents a particularly fascinating array of new behavioral methodologies as well as unique response categories altered by psychoactive agents, as well as emphasizing the highly relevant relationship between mechanisms of temperature regulation and the disposition and action of psychotropic agents. The role of genetic variables in determining the psychoactive effects of opiates, as detailed by Drs. Oliverio and Castellano, represents an important series of relationships between the basal chemical substrates upon which opiates act and changes that occur as a function of genetic differences. The implications for genetic bases of differences in tolerance, analgesic effects and addictive potential to opiates touches upon a variety of other issues to which the present chapter fundamentally relates.

In his chapter concerned with the behavioral effects of anticonvulsant drugs, Dr. Trimble highlights the behavioral effects and behavioral toxicity of these agents. The relevance of these drugs for psychiatric disorders represents an area too often overlooked—both in terms of therapeutic benefit as well as symptom exacerbation. There has been little said of anticonvulsant-psychotropic drug interactions on a behavioral or neurological level. The present chapter serves to clarify this issue. One issue of cardinal import to the clinician employing neuroleptic agents is their capacity to induce disorders of involuntary movements; such drug-induced tardive dyskinesia is the subject of Dr. Itoh's chapter in this volume. The mechanisms underlying tardive dyskinesia and how this entity differs from other movement disorders is clearly explicated. Moreover, attention to the prevention and treatment of tardive dyskinesia takes into account the mechanisms related to this entity as well as some of the bases for psychotropic drug action and central mechanisms for movement and movement disorders.

The prominence of smoking and the effects of nicotine in the scientific, clinical, as well as popular literature emphasizes the significance of the behavior and the drug across a broad spectrum of issues in health and disease. Questions regarding the why's of smoking behavior and the effects of nicotine have long concerned the researcher and the clinician. In their chapter on this subject, Drs. Kumar and Lader consider various aspects of nicotine in maintaining smoking behavior and how the behavioral effects, via brain mechanisms, relate to the behavioral consequences of exposure to this drug and how its re-exposure relates to its effects.

The anti-manic effects of lithium salts are well known and these agents have become well accepted in the psychiatric pharmacopae. The use of lithium salts in the treatment of depression, however, has not been as uniformly accepted, either as a therapeutic approach of particular advantage, or as a treatment modality for depression that is readily consistent with theoretical grounds. In their chapter Drs. Arieli and Lepkifker have provided a clinical-experimental framework within which the antidepressant actions of lithium are evaluated.

In the last chapter of this volume, Drs. Nagayama, Takagi, and Takahashi consider an important variable in the action of neuroleptic agents—the characteristics by which endogenous periodic variations provide for differences in their effects. Drug toxicity as well as behavioral efficacy appear to be regulated by the time period within which the drug is given and within which it is distributed, metabolized, and active. Both endogenous as well as exogenous regulatory mechanisms appear relevant to the onset, duration and efficacy of psychoactive drug effects, the basis for which may be sought on neurochemical, endocrinological, or neurophysiological bases, the interactions of which regulate the circadian influences upon drug action.

The seven chapters of this volume, although unique as far as chapters in prior volumes of this series are concerned, still constitute extensions of a continuum upon which the series was conceived, i.e., a comprehensive, yet contemporary, overview of the issues that comprise psychopharmacology. Although these issues have not fundamentally changed in the years since this series has been published, the variety of methodologies, the conceptual integration, and the psychopharmacopae have changed. This volume, while expanding the scope of subject coverage in the series, is also intended to serve the researcher and clinician as a perspective for issues of current focus and import for psychopharmacology.

The international scope of these volumes, represented by the roster of eminent contributors, has provided a rich resource of basic and clinical data. We thank the authors and we thank the members of the editorial advisory board who provided useful input and direction.

March, 1981                                                     Walter B. Essman
                                                               Flushing, N.Y.

                                                               Luigi Valzelli
                                                               Milan, Italy

# Contributors

**ARIEL ARIELI**
Sanatorium Hahlama Venofesh
Natanya, Israel

**CLAUDIO CASTELLANO**
Istituto di Psicobiologia e Psicofarmacologia,
   C.N.R.
Rome, Italy

**HITOSHI ITOH**
Department of Neuropsychiatry
School of Medicine, Keio University
Tokyo, Japan

**RAMESH KUMAR**
Department of Psychiatry
Institute of Psychiatry
University of London
London, England

**MALCOLM LADER**
Department of Psychiatry
Institute of Psychiatry
University of London
London, England

**KARI Y.H. LAGERSPETZ**
Zoophysiological Laboratory
Department of Biology
University of Turku
Turku, Finland

**ELIE LEPKIFKER**
Department of Psychiatry
Chaim Sheba Medical Center
Tel-Aviv University Medical School
Tel-Hashomer, Israel

**HARUO NAGAYAMA**
Department of Neuropsychiatry
Nagasaki University School of Medicine
Nagasaki, Japan

**ALBERTO OLIVERIO**
Istituto di Psicobiologia e Psicofarmacologia,
   C.N.R.
Rome, Italy

**AKINORI TAKAGI**
Department of Neuropsychiatry
Nagasaki University School of Medicine
Nagasaki, Japan

**RYO TAKAHASHI**
Department of Neuropsychiatry
Nagasaki University School of Medicine
Nagasaki, Japan

**MICHAEL TRIMBLE**
The National Hospitals for Nervous Diseases
London, England

# Contents

Current Developments in Psychopharmacology, Volume 6
© 1981, Spectrum Publications, Inc.

CHAPTER 1

# COMPARATIVE PSYCHOPHARMACOLOGY

## KARI Y.H. LAGERSPETZ

Abbreviations used in this chapter: A—adrenaline, epinephrine; ACh—acetylcholine; DA—dopamine; DNA—deoxyribonucleic acid; GABA—gamma-aminobutyric acid; 5-HT—5-hydroxytryptamine, serotonin; 5-HTP—5-hydroxytryptophan; L-DOPA—L-dehydroxyphenylalanine; LSD—$N,N$-diethyl-D-lysergamide; MAO—monoamino-oxidase; NA—noradrenaline, norepinephrine; p-CPA—para-chlorophenylalanine; RNA—ribonucleic acid.

## A. INTRODUCTION

### 1. Lower Animals as Models in Physiology and Pharmacology

There are about one million animal species living on the earth. More than 95 percent of them are poikilothermic, i.e., do not possess complicated thermoregulatory mechanisms. In birds and mammals, physiological thermoregulation makes the internal environment relatively constant in respect to one important physical variable—the temperature.

Conversely, more than 95 percent of pharmacological research is done on few homeothermic mammalian species, like the mouse, rat, guinea pig, rabbit, cat, dog, pig, and primates. These animals are regarded as closely enough related to man as to provide models of the human responses to chemical compounds. On the other hand, this concentration of the pharmacological work to relatively few species may leave certain experimental possibilities unexplored. During evolution, different organisms have acquired different solutions to overcome the problems encountered in their

1

environment. Therefore, "for many problems, there is an animal on which it can be most conveniently studied." This statement has been called the August Krogh Principle (Krebs, 1975) in honor of the Danish zoophysiologist and Nobel laureate August Krogh, whose work has given many examples of the solution of a biological problem by the choice of an appropriate test animal.

The importance and benefits of the study of different types of animals have long been recognized in physiology. There are many well-known examples in which the proper choice of the test animal has made an important advance possible. The nerve-muscle preparation of the frog has proved invaluable not only in the classical physiology of nerves and muscles, but also in the modern study of neuromuscular transmission. The discovery of the chemical transmission was done using the frog heart. Frog nerve fibers are used to study the mechanisms of saltatory conduction, and frog skin preparations to study the sodium transport mechanisms. Much of our present knowledge on the mechanism of nervous conduction is based on experiments on the giant nerve fibers of the squid, and other aspects of cellular neurophysiology have been successfully studied on the giant neurons of snails and slugs, as well as on the muscle receptors of the crayfish.

These examples show that so-called lower animals have often provided suitable preparations for the study of general physiological principles, and also, those fundamental to pharmacology. In addition to their use as models in general physiology, the study of lower animals has important comparative and evolutionary aspects. Comparative physiology and pharmacology attempt to relate the physiological and pharmacological differences found between species and other biological taxons to the ecology and evolutionary history of the taxons in question.

Like in this review, the term "comparative" is often used in a wider sense, to cover all studies pertaining to lower animals. In fact, during the 1970s, there has been a rise of interest in this wider meaning of comparative pharmacology. This is witnessed by the founding of the journals *Comparative and General Pharmacology* (1970; since 1975, published under the title *General Pharmacology*); and the Section C, *Comparative Pharmacology* (1975) of *Comparative Biochemistry and Physiology*; and by the publication of the two-volume treatise *Comparative Pharmacology*, edited by Michelson (1973). Much of the pertinent work continues to be published in a variety of pharmacological, physiological, biological, and psychological journals.

From time to time, reviews on different aspects of the pharmacology of invertebrates and poikilothermic vertebrates have been published (Crescitelli and Geissman, 1962; Fänge, 1962; Florey, 1965; Cottrell and Laverack, 1968; Baslow, 1969; Sakharov, 1970). And, an international symposium on comparative pharmacology was arranged in 1967 (*Federation Proceedings*, 1967). In the field of comparative neurophysiology, much attention has been paid to the occurrence and effects of neurotransmitters in poikilothermic animals (Bacq, 1947; Florey, 1961; Gerschenfeld, 1965, 1973; Murdock, 1971; Pitman, 1971; Kehoe and Marder, 1976).

Admitting the importance of the use of lower animal models in general pharmacology, we are justified to ask whether any contribution to psychopharmacology—to the understanding of the effects of chemical compounds on mind and behavior—is likely to come from such studies.

*Psychopharmaca* may be defined broadly as xenobiotic chemical compounds that affect the behavior and mental life through the central nervous system. The effects of such xenobiotic compounds as pesticides and antihelminth drugs are beyond the scope of this review, whether or not their action is mediated through the central nervous system of the target organism. So are the effects of hormones and pheromones; on the other hand, data on the effects of putative neurotransmitter substances on behavior are included, since many of the psychoactive drugs apparently exert their action by affecting chemical transmission.

One or more of the same neurotransmitter substances (ACh, A, NA, DA, 5-HT, and GABA) are known to occur in the nervous systems of most metazoan animals (Kehoe and Marder, 1976; Gerschenfeld, 1973); and even in some aneural organisms, e.g., protozoans (Lentz, 1968). It is therefore likely that many psychopharmaca that affect the metabolism, release, and uptake of neurotransmitters and/or their receptor molecules in man and other mammals would also be effective in producing changes in the central nervous system and behavior of other animals.

However, in spite of this relative chemical uniformity of the nervous systems that extends through the animal kingdom, the gross structural diversity of the nervous system is paralleled by the great variation in behavior. This brings us to the issue of how to define behavior and mental life, and to the problem of reductionism in neurosciences.

## 2. Dangers of Reductionism

In animal studies, behavior is commonly defined as the externally observable movement of an individual organism. It is perhaps even possible to subsume speech, the verbal behavior, under this concept. However, it is clear that such a concept is not relevant in psychopharmacology, since it leaves important targets of psychopharmaca unaccounted for, like states of mood, attentiveness, dreaming, and other states of consciousness. Such phenomena may occur not only in man, but also in other higher mammals.

The concept of behavior must also be broad enough to take into account those aspects of individual history that might appear as behavior modification. Learning and memory are in varying degree and scope present in all animals. The handling and storage of sensory information depends also on the previously stored information. Both clinical observations and animal experiments show that the deprivation of essential information about the environment leads to a failure in the development of some aspects of mental life. For man, as well as for some higher animals, social environment is very important in this respect.

Behavior can thus be conceived more broadly as mental life. According to this definition, mental life is a form of interaction between the organism and its environment; it consists of the externally observable movement of an individual organism and of the entire flow, handling, and storage of information in it, especially in its central nervous system. Although some of the general principles may be common to all types of centralized nervous systems, there is a large quantitative and qualitative variation between different animals in this flow and storage.

The behavior of lower animals, especially of invertebrates, shows less plasticity than that of mammals. The stereotypic behavioral patterns of lower animals can often be analyzed into simple behavioral responses. Some of these are likely to be common to a variety of animals, including higher mammals. On the other hand, certain complex forms of behavior occur only in these, and some are unique to man. Even the simple behavioral responses may be mediated by more complex mechanisms in the higher animals. The generalization to man of results obtained in studies with lower animals must therefore proceed with utmost caution.

In recent semipopular ethological literature, there have been many attempts to explain human behavior in terms used to explain the behavior of lower animals. The study of aggression has been especially contaminated by this type of reductive explanation. Scientists have become more concerned about the social problems of violence and war. An explanation offered by some ethologists and psychoanalysts is that aggressiveness is an inborn instinct—a drive in man like it is in some lower animals. If aggressiveness is a drive like thirst, hunger, and sexuality, it must always find an outlet, or become inhibited through severe punishment.

Even some animal studies show that this is not the case. Many different types of animals possess inborn nervous mechanisms that may mediate aggressive behavior, and the threshold values of these mechanisms show variation, which may, in part, be genetically determined. The presence of a nervous mechanism necessary for some kind of behavior does not, however, suffice to produce that kind of behavior. Even in mice, aggressiveness does not satisfy the criteria of a drive; it functions as a primary motive only when the aggressive state of the animal has been already aroused (Lagerspetz, 1964). As studies with man and mice show that aggressive behavior can be learned, results concerning the drive-like stereotypic aggression that is found in some lower animals should not be generalized.

One of the effects of ethyl alcohol in man is the notorious increase of aggressiveness. This effect has been interpreted as a release from the inhibitions against aggressive impulses. The effect of ethyl alcohol on aggressive behavior has also been studied in the Siamese fighting fish *Betta splendens*, the male of which is well known for its stereotypical aggressive behavior against other males of the same species and also against its own mirror image.

Raynes et al. (1968) studied the effects of the immersion of fighting fish in an ethyl alcohol solution (2.85 mg/ml) on the frequency of aggressive behavior directed against its mirror image and also on the learning not to approach another male through passive avoidance conditioning. The aggressive behavior pattern was more often displayed against its own mirror image under the effect of alcohol, and it was also more difficult to condition fish under alcohol not to approach another male. It has been shown that the blood alcohol in goldfish comes within 3 to 6 hours into equilibrium with the surrounding water, so that the fish can be studied at virtually constant blood alcohol levels (Ryback et al., 1969). The results of Raynes et al. (1968) appear to indicate that the aggressiveness of fighting fish is increased by alcohol as in man. Since fish do not have a developed neocortex, the authors suggest that this effect is produced at a subcortical level.

On the other hand, repeated attempts to produce aggressive behavior by alcohol administration in genetically aggressive mice with or without previous training to suppress aggression have been unsuccessful (Lagerspetz & Ekqvist, 1978). Ethyl alcohol even at low dose levels only depresses aggressive behavior; it never enhances it. These results seem to show that the aggression-increasing effect of alcohol cannot be a very general one, suppressing the inhibition of aggression in animals from fish to man.

This example may suffice to show the dangers of reductive explanations in psychopharmacology. Ethyl alcohol may weaken the socially learned inhibitions of aggressiveness in man; and it may act either as a painful stimulus eliciting aggression in fish immersed in it, or release some inhibitions of the brain stem mechanisms in them. However, it seems not to release the learned suppression of aggressiveness in mice. It is therefore difficult to think that the increases of aggressiveness in man and in the fighting fish caused by alcohol would depend on a similar mechanism.

It is clear that both reductive explanations and their opposite, anthropomorphic explanations should be avoided in research on animal behavior. However, when combined with careful interpretation of the results, behavioral experiments even on lower animals can be valuable contributions to psychopharmacology.

## 3. Variety of Approaches

Psychopharmaca are powerful tools for the modification of behavior and of the state of consciousness. One of the main reasons for giving such drugs to lower animals is to find out the action mechanisms of common psychoactive drugs; the use of poikilothermic animals in alcohol research is an example of this type of approach. Another impetus for comparative psychopharmacology comes from the need to find easy methods for the assessment of the type and intensity of behavioral effects of a chemical compound. This approach is important in behavioral toxicology and in the screening of possible psychopharmaca. The third reason for the administration of psychopharmaca to lower animals is, that by observing the effects of these drugs, it may be possible to learn something about the mechanisms of behavior. A thorough knowledge about the mechanisms of behavior of any animal cannot but help in the task of understanding human behavior and mental life.

The studies on the effects of drugs on the behavior of invertebrates and lower vertebrates can be subsumed under three categories: (1) studies on the action mechanisms of drugs, (2) studies aimed at the development of screening methods for psychopharmaca, and (3) studies on the mechanisms of behavior.

As complex as the behavior of animals is, only a few types of behavior have been studied as targets of psychopharmaca. (1) The spontaneous motor activity of animals is easy to observe and has therefore been the subject of many studies. In one case, this approach led to (2) the development of a screening test for antidepressant drugs.

Some of the stereotypic behavior patterns of lower animals have received special attention in the research reviewed here: (3) The effects of drugs on the web-building of spiders have been used for screening of psychopharmaca; (4) the attacks of a male Siamese fighting fish *Betta splendens* against a male of the same species or against its own mirror image have been used as a measure of the effects of different drugs on aggressiveness, as well as for the screening of psychopharmaca.

The effects of drugs on these and some other types of behavior have been studied as attempts to elucidate the mechanisms of behavior. This has been the main purpose of the studies on (5) the aggressive behavior in ants. In addition, (6) conditioning experiments both in fish and in (7) insect preparations have been performed, in order to study the mechanisms of learning and memory.

The majority of the psychopharmacological research done on poikilothermic animals belongs to one of the fields mentioned above. This work is reviewed on the following pages. Some of the studies on the effects of psychoactive drugs on other types of behavior are summarized at the end of this chapter.

## B.  SPONTANEOUS MOTOR ACTIVITY

### 1.  Cell Motility in Aneural Organisms

Some problems, partly semantical ones, are caused by the extreme broadness of many behavioral concepts. Spontaneous motor activity is one of these. The motor mechanisms of animals range from the pseudopodial, ciliary, and flagellar types of cell motility to complex muscular mechanisms. The latter are often controlled by the states of the central nervous system (CNS), e.g., by those controlling the circadian rhythms of rest and activity. Hence, the studies on motor activity exemplify the fact that it is often impossible to subsume behaviorally analogous phenomena found in different types of animals under a physiologically meaningful heading. Even the same chemical compounds may be critically involved in functions that are behaviorally analogous but very different in the complexity of their physiological mechanisms.

It is an interesting fact that cell motility is affected by neurochemical agents, like neurotransmitters and their antagonists. The pulsatory activity of the alternate contractions and expansions of the perikarya of cultured adult mammalian brain cells is accelerated by 5-HT (Geiger, 1963), as is also the phagocytosis of mammalian leucocytes (Ludány et al., 1958). Antagonists of 5-HT decrease the amoeboid motility of mesenchyme cells in the early embryo of sea urchin *Psammechinus miliaris*; while the motility can be restored by 5-HTP, which is the precursor of 5-HT (Gustafson and Toneby, 1970). According to Koshtoyants et al. (1961) and Gustafson et al. (1972), 5-HT also stimulates the ciliary activity and thus the motility of the embryos of marine gastropods and sea urchins.

ACh is another neurotransmitter that seems to affect cell motility. ACh stimulates the motility of sea urchin spermatozoa, while a specific acetylcholinesterase inhibitor (B.W. 284 C51 dibromide) reduces it (Nelson, 1972; Atherton, 1975). Antagonists of ACh also inhibit the contraction of pseudopods in the mesenchyme cells of the early sea urchin embryo (Gustafson and Toneby, 1970).

These and other examples, as well as the common occurrence of neurotransmitter substances in motile cells of various types, seem to indicate that these substances play a role in controlling the behavior of motile cells and aneural organisms. It is likely that this occurs through the effects of these substances on the cell membranes; definite membrane effects are associated with the motor activity and behavior of the ciliate *Paramecium* (Eckert, 1972).

Also, the sensitivity to stimuli in some aneural organisms is influenced by neurotropic drugs. Applewhite (1972) found that xylocaine, tubocurarine, strychnine, and indole acetic acid decreased the sensitvity of the ciliate *Spirostomum ambiguum* and the plant *Mimosa pudica* to mechanical stimuli; while ethyl alcohol, chlordiazepoxide (Librium), and caffeine were at the dose levels used without effect. The drugs used probably affected the membrane permeability in these two organisms by similar processes.

The facts that neurotransmitter substances are found in aneural motile organisms (Lentz, 1968), and that such compounds as well as neurotropic drugs affect the behavior of these organisms, indicate the generality of the molecular mechanisms controlling membrane permeability in all excitable cells. This idea has been originally put forward by Duncan (1967) in a stimulating monograph. In addition, these and other observations seem to point out that the phylogenetic and ontogenetic origin of the nervous system is to be sought in the primitive motile cells and their contacts.

## 2.  Spontaneous Motor Activity in Animals with a Nervous System

The effects of psychopharmaca on spontaneous motor activity have been studied in a number of metazoan animals of different phyla. Katona and Wolleman (1964) studied the effects of phenothiazines; these at relatively high concentrations reversibly inhibit the spontaneous movements in two coelenterates (a hydrozoan jellyfish and the sea anemone *Actinia equina*), in the medicinal leech *Hirudo medicinalis*, in the sea cucumber *Holothuria tubulosa*, and in the cephalopod *Octopus vulgaris*. The tranquilizers chlorpromazine and perphenazine are more potent than the antihistaminic sedative promethazine. The reactions to electric stimuli are either supressed or not affected.

When planarians (*Polycelis tenuis* and *Dugesia lugubris*) were immersed for 9 days into a solution of 8–10 $\mu$g/ml of reserpine, their motor activity was decreased and motor coordination impaired (Toğrol et al., 1966). Complete recovery from these effects took about 7 to 10 days. It is possible that the impairment of learning found in the conditioning and habituation experiments was also caused by the motor effects of reserpine. According to the review on primitive nervous systems by Lentz (1968), both catecholamines and 5-HT, as well as ACh and acetylcholinesterase, have been found to occur in coelenterates and in planarians.

The spontaneous motor activity of the carpenter ant *Camponotus herculeanus* and of the scorpion *Androctonus australis* is affected by a number of psychopharmaca (Cooper et al., 1971; Mercier and Dessaigne, 1970, 1971). The effects seen in the spontaneous spike activity of the cerebral ganglion of the scorpion are generally parallel to the motor effects (Goyffon et al., 1974). The injection of reserpine into the hemolymph results in an immobilization of the scorpion, and later in a complete disappearance of the spontaneous spike activity. This has been interpreted as an effect of the monoamine, especially 5-HT depletion, caused by reserpine.

Another arthropod, the house cricket *Acheta domesticus* exhibits a distinct diurnal rhythm of motor activity. Both reserpine and LSD reduce the level of motor activity and abolish its rhythmicity, while 5-HT increases the activity level (Cymborowski, 1970). Reserpine also reduces motor activity of the flour beetle *Tribolium confusum* (Huot et al., 1960).

In mollusks, the activity of fresh water mussels *Anodonta cygnea* is increased by 5-HT, 5-HTP, and also by reserpine; while p-CPA decreases it, and the MAO inhibitors actomol and nialamide, as well as α-methyl-DOPA, are without effect (Hiripi and Salánki, 1973). The authors conclude that 5-HT processes maintain the rhythmic activity in this mussel. The observations by Abramson and Jarvik (1955) and Jarvik (1957), according to which the motor activity of the snails *Physa* and *Ampullaria cuprina* is disturbed by fairly low concentrations of LSD, may also point out to the importance of 5-HT neurons in the maintenance of normal motor activity in mollusks. The observations of Mirolli and Welsh (1964) on a variety of mollusk species are also in agreement with this concept. In a number of mollusks, both reserpine and LSD affect the spontaneous activity—reserpine by increasing the tonus of the smooth muscles around the large peripheral hemolymph lacunae, and LSD by decreasing it. In addition, reserpine abolishes the tonus of the shell muscles. Reserpine also depletes the 5-HT stores in the ganglia. The time course of this effect is temperature-dependent.

While some evidence thus seems to point out the importance of 5-HT processes for the spontaneous motor activity of arthropods and mollusks, the results obtained in experiments with lower vertebrates are different. Intramuscularly injected 5-HT inhibits spontaneous motor activity in the goldfish, while LSD counteracts this effect (Sacchi and Gianniotti, 1956a, 1956b). In the killifish *Fundulus grandis*, in which serotonergic mechanisms apparently participate in the maintenance of the circadian rhythm, 5-HT decreases motor activity (Fingerman, 1976). In amphibians, application of 5-HT into the lymph sac on brain surface produces a deep sedation in the frog *Rana esculenta* (Dolce and Garello, 1956), a fact to which we will return presently.

In the tortoise *Testudo graeca*, reserpine produces a large decrease in the catecholamine concentrations, especially in DA concentrations in different parts of the brain (Juorio, 1973). However, no changes in the gross behavior of the tortoises have been observed. In another reptile, the South American caiman *Caiman sclerops*, reserpine progressively decreased the brain levels of catecholamines and 5-HT, but did not affect the motor activity of the animals (Doshi and Huggins, 1977). When an administration of 6-hydroxydopamine followed a pretreatment with desmethylimipramine, DA was the only monoamine significantly depleted. The motor activity was also reduced. This suggests the importance of DA neurons for the motor functions in the caiman.

A few words about the methods used for the induction of immobility and general anesthesia in poikilothermic animals may be in place. In aquatic invertebrates, magnesium salts, ethyl urethane, ethyl alcohol, and later also tricaine methanesulfonate (MS 222; methanesulfonate of *m*-aminobenzoic acid ethyl ester) have been used for anesthesia. In insects, diethyl ether and carbon dioxide have been the anesthetics of choice.

Surprisingly, there seem to be rather few systematical studies on the effects of anesthetics in lower vertebrates. Cherkin and Catchpool (1964) studied the effect of temperatures between 5 and 30 C on the anesthetic partial pressure of the volatile anesthetics diethyl ether, chloroform, halothane, and methoxyflurane in goldfish. The concentrations of the drugs in water, which anesthetized 50 percent of the fish, decreased in the above order. The corresponding partial pressures increased linearly from 10 to 30 C.

After its introduction, MS-222 has rapidly become the anesthetic most used for lower vertebrates. Its effects have been studied in some detail (Stenger and Maren, 1974; Houston and Woods, 1976; Ohr, 1976a, 1976b). MS-222 is to be used preferably as a neutralized solution (Smit and Hattingh, 1979).

## C. SEDATION IN THE FROG: A SCREENING TEST FOR TYMOLEPTICS

The concentration of NA in different areas of the brains of frogs *Rana pipiens*, *R. temporaria*, *Hyla cinerea* is much lower than in mammals and also lower than that of A (Brodie and Bogdanski, 1964; Harri, 1972b; Juorio, 1973). It is possible that the adrenergic mechanisms are of minor importance in the central control of behavioral arousal in frogs, compared with most other vertebrates. While reserpine does not produce any clear action on the motor behavior of the frog (Brodie and Bogdanski, 1964), after a pretreatment with the MAO inhibitor pargyline, it has a sedative effect, paralleled by a rise in the brain 5-HT level but by only a slight change in the brain A level. Brodie and Bogdanski (1964) thus suggest that the sedative action of reserpine is due to the accumulation of free 5-HT, stabilized by the blockade of MAO. This suggestion is in agreement with the results of Dolce and Garello (1956), the authors who reported the sedative action of 5-HT applied into a lymph sac brought into contact with the brain surface.

The tricyclic antidepressants imipramine and desmethylimipramine potentiate the sedative effect of a combined MAO inhibitor and reserpine or 5-HTP treatment in the frog *Rana temporaria* (Lapin et al., 1968). On the basis of this result, as well on a large amount of research on the peripheral and central effects of 5-HT processes in mammals, Lapin and Oxenkrug (1969) suggested that the mechanism of the mood-elevating action of tricyclic antidepressants would mainly be the potentiation of the effects of 5-HT, while psychic depression may be a result of brain 5-HT deficiency. Apart from this, the activation of central catecholaminergic mechanisms by antidepressants would account for the stimulation of motor activity observed.

Lapin et al. (1970) also suggested the potentiation of the reserpine sedation in the frog, measured as the loss of the righting reflex, and the occurrence of muscle twitches in the limbs to be used as a test for screening possible antidepressant drugs. Tricyclic antidepressants had these effects, while neuroleptics, anticholinergic drugs, and amphetamine did not enhance the effects of reserpine. Even at high dose levels, chlorpromazine and benactyzine increased only the sedative effect. Dimethyl tricyclic antidepressants were more effective in this test than their monomethyl derivatives (Oxenkrug and Lapin, 1971). This difference was not related to the effectiveness of these drugs to produce sedation without pretreatment by a MAO inhibitor and reserpine.

The brain level of 5-HT is lower in frogs in winter than in summer, but the depletion of 5-HT after the inhibition of its biosynthesis by p-CPA is larger in winter, thus indicating a higher activity of 5-HT neurons in the winter conditions studied (Harri, 1972a). In winter, the frogs were also more sensitive to the sedative action of imipramine (Harri, 1974), which shows that not only drugs, but environmental conditions that physiologically alter the release of 5-HT, affect the sedative effect of antidepressants. The test of Lapin et al. (1970) may therefore be used not only for screening of possible antidepressants, but conversely, to measure the central serotonergic activity in frogs.

## D.  WEB-BUILDING IN SPIDERS

A number of spiders perform from time to time (some of them every morning) a complicated behavior pattern, which results in the construction of a web for the capture of prey animals. The webs of the orb-web type are built in one plane and are bilaterally or even radially symmetrical. A web built by an adult female cross spider contains about 0.1 to 0.5 mg of silk material secreted by specific glands, spun to 10 to 20 m of thread with 1000 to 2000 fused crossings. It is completed in 20 to 30 minutes (Witt, 1971).

When attempting to shift the usual time of web-building from the time just before sunrise to another time of the day, Peters and Witt (1949) made the accidental observation that psychostimulant drugs altered the usual geometrical pattern of the webs and also the web-building frequency. This finding initiated a series of studies by Witt and his co-workers on the effects of psychoactive and other drugs on the web-building of spiders and the development of a screening test for psychopharmaca. This work represents an early and original contribution to the behavioral pharmacology of invertebrates. As this research has been extensively reviewed by its originator (Witt, 1956; Witt et al., 1968; Witt, 1971), only a brief summary of it is given here.

The species most used in this research are the cross spider *Araneus diadematus* and *Zygiella x-notata*. The effects observed seem to be common for several species studied. Most of the drugs are ingested by spiders by drinking drops of water also containing sugar.

Methamphetamine was one of the first psychoactive drugs tested (Peters and Witt, 1949; Peters et al., 1950; Wolff and Hempel, 1951), and these tests have since been repeated with similar results also with d-amphetamine. Amphetamine decreases the web-building frequency and the size of the webs. It also distorts the usual regularity of the angles between the radial threads and of the distances between the different turns of the spiral thread. The concentration-dependency of the effect is seen both in the web-building frequency and in the duration of the effects on the web pattern, which for high doses may last up to 4 days after the administration of the drug (Wolff and Hempel, 1951; Witt, 1971).

The MAO inhibitor iproniazid, which by itself does not affect the web-building, prolongs and enhances the effects of amphetamine. Iproniazid also inhibits the catabolism of amphetamine and delays its disappearance from the body of the spiders (Witt et al. 1961). Another antidepressant, imipramine, has no known effect on web-building and also fails to affect the behavioral effects and catabolism of amphetamine in the spider. This test therefore seems to differentiate between tricyclic antidepressants and such of the MAO inhibitor type.

Many other psychoactive drugs, like chlorpromazine, diazepam, and psilocybin reduce the frequency of web-building (Witt, 1955; Christiansen et al., 1962; Reed and Witt, 1968). Diazepam and phenobarbital reduce the size of the web and cause some irregularity of its pattern, apparently decreasing the motor activity of the spiders (Reed and Witt, 1968). Astonishingly, LSD increases the regularity of the web (Witt, 1951; Groh and Lemieuz, 1968); while another hallucinogen, mescaline, reduces its regularity (Christiansen et al., 1962). Extremely distorted webs are built after ingestion of high doses of caffeine (Witt, 1971).

The complexity of the web-building performance makes many different drug-induced variations possible. It is of interest whether any factors active in this test can be found in the body fluids of mental patients. In spite of attempts by Witt and other laboratories, no such biologically active compounds have been discovered (Witt, 1971). The studies on the psychopharmacology of the web-building in spiders show, that even the stereotyped behavior of invertebrates may be very complex and may be affected, often in a specific way, by a number of psychopharmaca.

The spinning behavior of the larva of the silk moth *Bombyx mori*, when building its cocoon, is the basis of the ancient and still important silk industry. Tamano (1960) studied the effects of some neurotropic drugs and mitose inhibitors on cocoon building. It is remarkable that this well-known stereotypic behavior of an insect has apparently not been subject to other pharmacological research.

## E.  AGGRESSIVE BEHAVIOR

### 1.  Aggressive Behavior in Ants

Kostowski et al. (1965, 1966) studied the effects of several neurotropic and psychotropic drugs on the motor activity, phototropic response, and spontaneous electrical activity (EEG) of the optical lobes in the wood ant *Formica rufa.* Reserpine either alone, or 12 hours after nialamide, inhibited the motor activity of the ants, but also produced outbursts of aggressive behavior. Chlorpromazine both inhibited motor activity and caused disturbances of motor coordination, but did not provoke aggressive behaviour. LSD did not affect the behavior but the EEG was slightly changed. Clordiazepoxide and amphetamine were without effects.

The observation that reserpine induces aggressive behavior in the wood ant has led Kostowski and his co-workers to a series of studies on the effects of neurohormones and psychopharmaca on aggressive behavior. Both interspecific aggression, appearing as attacks against a beetle, and intraspecific aggression, directed towards members of its own species, have been studied. Intraspecific aggression has been observed either in a fight situation with a beetle or after antennectomy, which apparently destroys the olfactory capacity of ants (Vowles, 1964).

Reserpine and LSD decreased interspecific aggressiveness in ants after 2 to 3 hours; but in 18 to 24 hours after drug administration, aggressiveness was increased (Kostowski, 1966). Amphetamine, phenobarbitone, chlordiazepoxide, and chlorpromazine did not affect the interspecific aggressiveness. Of anticholinergic drugs, atropine and scopolamine decreased both interspecific aggressiveness and electric activity of the optical lobes, while tubocurarine had opposite effects (Kostowski, 1968). Although 5-HT and 5-HTP decreased interspecific aggressive behavior, they increased mutual, intraspecific aggressiveness. In connection with this, the amplitude of the EEG activity from optical lobes was also increased (Kostowski and Tarchalska, 1972). LSD again decreased both aggressiveness and the EEG amplitude.

These studies by Kostowski and his co-workers have, besides giving data on the effects of psychopharmaca in ants, mainly attempted to find out the neurochemical mechanisms of aggressive behavior in these insects. Consequently, Tarchalska et al. (1975) and Kostowski et al. (1975a) studied the effects of fights with a beetle or with other ants on the concentrations of 5-HT, NA, and A in the cerebral ganglion. The levels of 5-HT and A were increased, and the level of NA decreased by the fights, but also to a lesser amount by the transfer of the ants from their nest to the experimental conditions. These effects may therefore, in part, be caused by non-specific stress caused by the handling of the animals and their transfer out of the nest.

In addition, DA, L-DOPA, and the DA hydroxylase inhibitor diethyl-dithiocarbamate (DDTC) increased intraspecific aggression in ants, but did not change the aggressive behavior toward other species (Kostowski et al., 1975b). Both DA and L-DOPA decreased the amplitude of EEG and the spontaneous activity of neurons in the protocerebrum, while DDTC and L-DOPA increased the concentrations of A and DA in the cerebral ganglion. On the other hand, haloperidol decreased the intraspecific aggressive behavior and motor activity, but did not seem to affect the EEG or neuronal activity.

This work shows, that, even in ants, monoamines are involved in the mediation of aggressive behavior and probably also of stress effects. Specific parallels between mammals and ants are difficult to draw, partly because the research on mammals has paid less attention to the immediate effects of fight than to the neurochemical concomitants of aggressiveness. Fighting and stress seem to increase the 5-HT levels in the central nervous system (CNS) of both mammals (Welch and Welch, 1968) and ants; on the other hand, high 5-HT turnover is associated with low tendency to aggressive behavior in mammals (Valzelli, 1974). Increased catecholamine levels or turnover rates again generally seem to be associated with high aggressiveness.

## 2.  Aggressive Behavior in Fish

Males of many fish species show stereotypic aggressive behavior against other males of the same species, some also against their own mirror image. The Siamese fighting fish *Betta splendens* is the most well-known of these. Its attacks are preceded by a display consisting of deepening coloration, erection of the gill cover, as well as extensions of fins. The convict cichlid *Cichlasoma nigrofasciatum* is another species, the territorial aggressiveness of which makes it suitable for psychopharmacological studies (Peeke et al., 1975).

The fish seem to be advantageous as experimental animals in behavioral pharmacology, since the drugs to be tested can be dissolved in the water of the test aquaria and need not to be injected. This rests on the assumption that drugs will enter from the surrounding water to the blood of the fish. As the gills of fish are permeable to oxygen, carbon dioxide, some ions, and other substances, this assumption is not unreasonable, although for most drugs it is unproved. In goldfish, the blood alcohol level comes within 3 to 6 hours into equilibrium with the alcohol concentration in the surrounding water, so the goldfish can be studied at virtually constant blood alcohol levels (Ryback et al., 1969; Ryback, 1970). Peeke et al. (1973) showed that the blood alcohol level of convict cichlids *Cichlasoma nigrofasciatum* rises in about 2 hours to a level corresponding to about one half of the alcohol concentration in the surrounding water, and is stabilized to a level of about two thirds of it in about 6 hours.

Only a few drugs have been studied in this respect. The movement across the gills of fish and the general pharmacokinetics of the anesthetic MS-222 are rather well-known both in fish and in amphibians (Hunn and Allen, 1974; Stenger and Maren, 1974; Houston and Woods, 1976; Ohr, 1976a, 1976b). The studies on the absorption of another fish anesthetic, quinaldine, and of a lampricide, 3-trifluormethyl-4-nitrophenol have been also reviewed by Hunn and Allen (1974).

However, there is a specific problem concerning the fishes of the Anabantid family, to which the Siamese fighting fish belongs. These fish are predominantly air-breathing; and therefore, as Figler (1973) points out, probably absorb drugs slower than fish breathing with gills.

Abramson and Evans (1954) and Abramson (1957) were the first to study the effects of the psychoactive drug, LSD, on the behavior of the Siamese fighting fish. When the fish were immersed for several hours in water containing LSD, even concentrations as low as 0.1 $\mu$g/ml produced observable symptoms. LSD inhibited motor activity and disturbed the motor coordination, causing a stupor-like state in the fish, as well as a suppression of aggressive behavior. However, the immersion of female Siamese fighting fish in water solution containing LSD clearly increased their aggressive behavior (Evans et al., 1958). Evans and co-workers also compared the behavioral effects of LSD with eight other ergot derivatives, mescaline, and meperidine hydrochloride (Evans et al., 1956). From these, only LSD produced the typical loss of the control of trunk musculature and quiescence, which may last for days after an immersion of the fishes for 4 hours in the LSD solution. When compared with other ergot derivatives, LSD seems hence to have specific effects not only in man but also in the fighting fish, and in the guppy *Lebistes reticulatus (Poecilia reticulata)* (Keller and Umbreit, 1956). The latter authors also found that long-lasting abnormal behavior caused by LSD in the fighting fish could be returned to normal by reserpine.

Besides LSD and mescaline, *Cannabis* hallucinogens have also been tested on the aggressive behavior of Siamese fighting fish. Marihuana extract and $\Delta^9$-tetrahydrocannabinol (0.5–1 $\mu$g/ml) suppressed aggressive behavior. Motor activity was also slightly depressed, but not the motor coordination. A tolerance to the effect of these hallucinogens was developed after 9 exposures of 2 hours each (González et al., 1971).

Walaszek and Abood (1956) studied the effects of different types of psychopharmaca on the motor activity and fighting response of the fighting fish. Reserpine and meprobamate (10 $\mu$g/ml in water) inhibited the aggressive display without apparent impairment of the motor activity, while chlorpromazine (2 $\mu$g/ml) and barbiturates (20–30 $\mu$g/ml) produced sedation. The barbiturates at these concentrations did not prevent threat responses against normal males, but inhibited continued attack behavior. Antihistamine drugs inhibited aggressive responses as well as the motor activity, to a varying degree. The effects of tranquilizers are obviously temperature-dependent, since reserpine and chlorpromazine (4 $\mu$g/ml) abolished the fighting response at water temperatures of 14–20 C and 30–38 C, but not at the intermediate temperature range (20–30 C) (Cano Puerta, 1959). The mechanism of this interaction between temperature and drug effects still remains unexplained.

A number of attempts have been made in order to find out whether the effects on the behavior of the Siamese fighting fish can be used to differentiate between types of psychopharmaca. Boissier and Pagny (1959) found in tests with a number of major and minor tranquilizers and hypnotics behavioral effects that were clearly different for the studied groups and subgroups of psychopharmaca. However, Boissier and Pagny used several behavioral variables, and not only fighting and aggressive display to assess the effects of drugs. Oelkers (1960) did not find the fighting test suitable to differentiate between the effects of chlorpromazine, promazine, meprobamate, and barbiturates, although most of them attenuate attack behavior at concentrations not affecting motor activity (for secobarbital, see also Figler and Bennett, 1974).

Obviously, for general screening purposes, the observation of only a single type of behavior like aggression can seldom be sufficient. The more behavioral features that can be reliably observed in a test, the more valid are the differences and similarities found.

On the other hand, psychopharmaca may be used to study the relations of different types of behavior to each other and to demonstrate differences and similarities in their mechanisms.

Chlordiazepoxide (Librium) decreased the aggressive behavior against another male fighting fish and also facilitated its habituation without any sedative effect. On the other hand, some components of normal sexual behavior were directed against the male partner (Figler, 1973; Figler et al., 1975). This points out that the mutually inhibitory relationship between sexual and aggressive behavior which has been found in mice (Lagerspetz and Hautojärvi, 1967) may also occur in fish.

Morphine (5–10 $\mu$g/ml) did not affect the predatory behavior of the convict cichlid, as measured by the latency to ingest 10 out of 12 living brine shrimps, but decreased the frequency of aggressive displays directed towards another male of the same species (Avis and Peeke, 1975). This indicates that the central mechanisms of predation and intraspecific aggression are different as are the specificity of the effects of morphine. However, in the Siamese fighting fish, morphine (40 µg/ml) rather enhanced the intraspecific aggressiveness (Walaszek and Abood, 1956).

It is interesting that Siamese fighting fish seem to be able to associate the increased aggressive display caused by morphine as well as the depression of aggressive behavior caused by the antihistaminic sedative promethazine with neutral stimuli, such as flickering lights of different color. In the experiments of Braud and Weibel (1969), the stimuli used continued to affect aggressive display directed toward the mirror image of the fish specifically, even after the drug administration was discontinued.

The effects of ethyl alcohol on the aggression in fish have, for the most part, documented the biphasic concentration effect of alcohol: psychostimulatory at low concentrations and sedative at high concentrations. Ethyl alcohol at a low concentration (2.85 mg/ml) prolongs the attack behavior of the Siamese fighting fish during passive avoidance conditioning and also increases the frequency of gill displays evoked by its own mirror image, while a higher concentration (6.5 mg/ml) inhibits the latter behavior (Raynes et al., 1968). Both bourbon whisky, diluted to give the low and stimulatory alcohol concentration, and a corresponding dilution of the congener substances present in bourbon, actually decrease the time of gill displays directed to the mirror image (Raynes and Ryback, 1970). Apparently, the mechanisms of the effects of alcohol and the congeners are not the same.

Peeke et al. (1973) have studied the effects of ethyl alcohol on attacks of convict cichlids against a conspecific male. Alcohol (1.8–3.3 mg/ml) inhibits attacks but causes no motor disturbances. Those fish that make attacks in the alcohol solution show increased display frequency and time, as well as biting frequency at 1.8 mg/ml, but greatly decreased values of these parameters at 3.3 mg/ml of alcohol. The later results of Peeke et al. (1975) confirm this biphasic action of alcohol, low concentrations causing hyperaggressiveness, and high hypoaggressiveness in this fish species. However, these results must be interpreted with caution. Low alcohol concentrations may act as painful unspecific irritants, while high concentrations are sedative.

Compared with the studies in mammals and ants, the monoamine hypotheses of aggressive behavior have not been tested very much on fish. Immersion in water containing NA increased the occurrence of spontaneous fin extension and deepening of the gill coloration (Marrone et al., 1966), but conversely, both NA and A inhibited the aggressive displays of the Siamese fighting fish to its own mirror image (Baenninger, 1968). There were large interindividual differences in the reactivity to catecholamines. Those less affected by catecholamines were also usually most dominant in groups of five fish, but not in paired encounters. The behavior of dominant fish could be changed by A to resemble that of the submissive ones in other respects, except in chasing the opponents. On the other hand, D-amphetamine (2 mg/l) increased the aggressiveness of Siamese fighting fish against their mirror images or artificial decoys (Weischer, 1966).

During the last 25 years, lithium has been widely used in the treatment of recurrent affective disorders, like those connected with mania, aggressiveness, and addiction. Lithium chloride (0.4–1.3 mg/ml in surrounding water) in 7–24 hours reversibly inhibited the fighting behavior of *Betta splendens* (Weischer, 1969), and in 6 hours reduced social aggregation (schooling) in the goldfish (Johnson, 1979). These treatments did not affect the motor activity of either species. Lithium thus probably impairs the central processing of sensory stimuli necessary for social responses in fish (Johnson, 1979).

## F.  LEARNING AND MEMORY

The often stereotyped behavior patterns of lower animals are, however, affected by many ambient environmental conditions. Some types of behavior can also be more permanently, but reversibly, modified by repeating the releasing stimuli either alone or in combination with other stimuli. Different types of learning and memory represent instances of this plasticity of behavior found in all animals. Studies on the effects of drugs on learning and memory may elucidate their mechanisms; they may also be of practical importance in the treatment of amnesias and in the maintenance of memory and learning capacity in the aged.

The interest in the study of the biological and molecular basis of learning and memory was stimulated by the discoveries concerning the structure of DNA and the main steps involved in the protein synthesis in the 1950s and early 1960s. As these findings showed how the genetic information was coded and read out, attempts were made to find analogous solutions to the problems of storage and decoding of information in the brain. Most of this work has been done on laboratory mammals. However, especially insects and fish have been to some extent used in the study of the effects of drugs on learning and memory.

### 1.  Learning and Memory in Insects

Insect models suitable for studies on learning are the headless cockroach *Periplaneta americana* preparation, introduced by Horridge (1962), and the isolated segment preparation from the cockroach (Eisenstein and Cohen, 1965). The latter contains only a single ganglion, but shows similar learning properties as the headless cockroach. Eisenstein (1965) was the first to use this method to demonstrate the effects of drugs (strychnine and pentobarbital) on learning.

The learning paradigm used in these experiments with insect models is shock-avoidance conditioning (Figure 1). The preparation to be trained and its control preparation are connected in a series with an electric stimulator and a saline contactor. Each time the leg attached to the preparation to be trained lowers enough to make a contact through the saline, both preparations receive a shock. In the preparation to be trained, this depends on the position of the leg; in the yoked control preparation there is no such relation. When retested for the possible retention of training effects, the preparations are coupled in parallel with the stimulator. Now both preparations receive a shock separately when their own legs touch the saline. This occurs much less often for the trained preparation, which has learned to keep its leg raised.

It would, of course, be interesting to know whether specific RNA or protein synthesis is necessary for learning. This problem has been studied by using a protein synthesis inhibitor, cycloheximide, and an RNA synthesis inhibitor, actinomycin D (Brown and Noble, 1967, 1968; Glassman et al., 1970). Both of these putative learning inhibitors also seem to have an unspecific effect of stimulating the leg activity. This seems to explain their apparent inhibitory effects on learning in this preparation (Eisenstein, 1968; Glassman et al., 1970). Also yoked controls were not used in these experiments.

As Eisenstein (1968) has pointed out, this learning paradigm has an obvious and not uncommon drawback in its use for drug studies: Any drug increasing the "spontaneous" activity of the effector (the leg) would seem to inhibit avoidance learning, since it interferes with the quiet state of the leg in the raised position, which is necessary for avoiding shocks. The results obtained with these models must therefore be interpreted with caution.

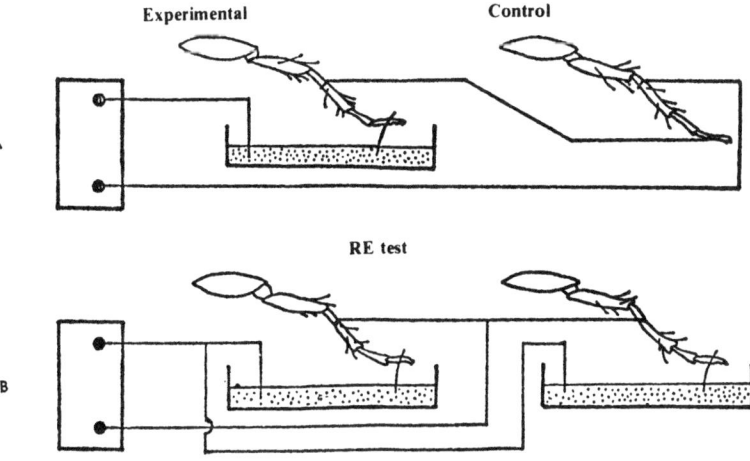

**Figure 1.**   Training and retesting circuits used for avoidance conditioning of cockroach preparations (Horridge, 1962; Kerkut et al., 1970).

Kerkut et al. (1970) reported that, among other drugs, cycloheximide and actinomycin D inhibited learning, while amphetamine, prostigmine, and magnesium pemoline facilitated it. On the other hand, the level of the cholinesterase activity in the ganglion was inversely related with the avoidance behavior. The increase of shock avoidance produced by conditioning might also be associated with a higher level of GABA (Leake and Taylor, 1972).

It is perhaps safe to say that the initial interest evoked by the introduction of insect preparations to the study of the psychopharmacology of learning has waned in the mid-1970s. One reason for this is probably the excellent analysis of relevant problems by Eisenstein (1968), which shows that even this approach is not simple, although promising. Lovell and Eisenstein (1973) have also introduced another method to study avoidance learning in cockroach, dark-avoidance conditioning. Carbon dioxide seems to disrupt memory formation if administered immediately after training, but not if given 1 hour later. Different phases in the memory formation in the cockroach have different susceptibilities to carbon dioxide; this may also be true for psychoactive drugs.

## 2.  Learning and Memory in Fishes

### a.  Effects of Compounds Affecting the Biosyntheses of Proteins and RNA

Fishes, especially the goldfish, have been used extensively in studies concerning learning and memory. Most of the studies on drug effects have attempted to clarify the possible role of the synthesis of RNA and proteins in the memory formation, and the drugs used have therefore been known to inhibit these syntheses (Agranoff and Davis, 1968; Laudien, 1977a). Learning in goldfish has also provided a suitable model for the study of amnesia caused by ethyl alcohol (Ryback, 1969b). In addition, a number of psychoactive drugs have been tested for their ability to affect learning and memory in fishes.

Goldfish can be trained to avoid electric shocks by swimming over a barrier upon a light signal (Horner et al., 1961). This is an example of the learning paradigm called active avoidance conditioning. It is often used in studies with rats and mice. The apparatus used is called a shuttle box (Figure 2). Goldfish increase their avoidance performance during 20 training trials given in 40 minutes, and some retention of the training can be seen in retraining trials 3 days later (Agranoff and Klinger, 1964; Davis et al., 1965).

An intracranial injection of puromycin, an inhibitor of protein synthesis, given within 1 hour after training trials, impairs the retention from the training progressively during 3 days (Agranoff and Klinger, 1964; Davis et al., 1965; Davis and Agranoff, 1966; Agranoff et al., 1965). Puromycin

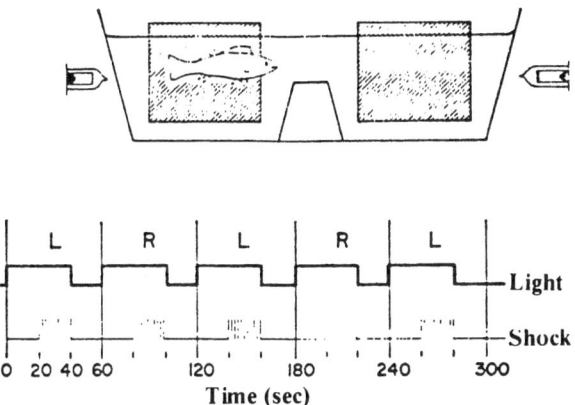

**Figure 2.** Diagram of shuttle box for goldfish with lights and grid electrodes for shocks on both sides of an underwater barrier to be crossed. Below is a diagram of a trial sequence in which light is turned on (or off) and the fish shocked alternately in the left (L) and the right (R) compartments (Agranoff et al., 1966).

injected before the training trials does not have this effect. Agranoff and co-workers have suggested that puromycin especially affects the process of memory fixation.

These studies have been repeated and extended by Agranoff's group and also in other laboratories. Potts and Bitterman (1967) tried to answer the question of whether the effect of puromycin is to interfere with the memory of the conditioned fear rather than with the memory of the performance itself. These authors trained goldfish to avoid electric shock preceded either by a green or an amber light signal. The signal of the other color was not followed by shock. The fish injected intracranially with puromycin immediately after each of the 6 training sessions given 1 week apart showed less increase in their avoidance performance than those injected with saline or with puromycin 24 hours after training. In each case, fish showed more avoidance responses to light signals paired with electric shocks than to the signals alone, but puromycin injected immediately after training impaired the avoidance performance in both types of experiments. These results could be interpreted as an interference with the conditioned fear.

Potts and Bitterman (1967) trained other groups of fish for a number of days in a runway to swim to a goal box with a food reward. At the last trial, the fish received electric shocks for 30 seconds in the goal box instead of food. After this they were immediately injected with puromycin or with saline. One week later, the mean swimming time to the goal box with reward was shorter in fish that had received puromycin. This seems to show that puromycin does not interfere with the performance, but with the consolidation of conditioned fear. This means that in the avoidance experiments, fish would fail to avoid because the conditioned stimulus (light signal) would not elicit fear in the puromycin group.

On the other hand, Schoel and Agranoff (1972) conditioned the deceleration of the heart rate of goldfish to a light-off signal paired with an electric shock. Injection of puromycin immediately before or after the training session did not block the formation of memory of this response. If the deceleration of the heart rate is interpreted as an autonomic response related to fear or attentiveness, puromycin did not apparently interfere with the retention of these.

The effects of other inhibitors of protein synthesis on the learning and memory of fishes have also been tested. Acetoxycycloheximide blocks the memory formation in an avoidance learning task (Agranoff et al., 1966; Agranoff and Davis, 1968). The inhibitors of RNA synthesis, actinomycin D (Agranoff et al., 1967), and camptothecin (Neale et al., 1973a) also block the memory of conditioned avoidance in the goldfish; while an inhibitor of DNA synthesis, cytosine arabinoside, is not effective in this respect (Casola et al., 1968).

One of the general results of the studies on the effects of these inhibitors on learning and memory is the time-dependency of the effectiveness of these drugs. Retention of a conditioned shock-avoidance response is decreased if the inhibitors are administered to fish shortly after conditioning. They are without effect when given a few hours or days after the initial training (Springer and Agranoff, 1976). The period of the susceptibility to puromycin is affected by temperature (Neale et al., 1973b): The effect of puromycin on memory is decreased if the fish are kept at 30 C for a period of 90 minutes between the training and drug injection at 20 C. Cooling of the fish to 4.5 C for 24 hours after the training session impairs the memory. These results are interpreted to show that there is a phase of memory consolidation through protein synthesis. The impairment of RNA synthesis with actinomycin D blocks the fixation of long-time memory also in passive avoidance conditioning experiments in goldfish (Ohi, 1975).

An important step in these studies would obviously be the demonstration of changes in the composition of brain RNA related to learning, although any major changes in it may be considered *a priori* improbable because of the relatively small role of the recently acquired modification of behavior in the total behavioral repertoire and other possibly RNA-coded functions of the animal. A study on the effect of learning on the RNA-base ratios in the brain was done by Shashoua (1968a, 1968b).

When a foam polystyrene float is attached to the ventral surface of a goldfish, this initially disturbs its swimming position; but within 2 to 3 hours the animal learns to swim horizontally in spite of the float. Fish injected with puromycin prior to the training do not differ from the controls in the acquisition of the new performance, but in contrast to the control fish, show no retention of it when retested with the float after 22 hours. The uridine/cytosine ratio of the brain RNA is changed by the training, except in the puromycin group, which also shows no retention (Shashoua, 1968a, 1968b). In this experiment, the changes in the RNA-base ratios seem to be related to learning, but stress effects on protein synthesis attenuated by puromycin cannot be ruled out.

All these experiments on the effects of putative memory-blocking drugs on fish have been based on the paradigm of avoidance conditioning with electric shocks as punishment. If these substances do affect the memory of specific tasks rather than that of conditioned fear, they should also block the memory of the extinction of learned avoidance performance, as well as the memory of tasks learned through positive reinforcement. In an experiment of Braud and Broussard (1973), puromycin injections given immediately after extinction sessions without shock actually inhibited the effect of extinction on the previously acquired avoidance behavior. The frequency of avoidance responses was not decreased in the fish that had received puromycin immediately after the extinction sessions.

Unexpectedly, paradigms of positive reinforcement through rewards have not been much used in studies on the effects of drugs on the learning and memory in fishes. Batkin et al. (1966) studied the effects of intracranial injections of puromycin, actinomycin D, and RNA on the acquisition and retention by carps *Cyprinus carpio* of a positively reinforced visual discrimination task presented in a T-maze. Actinomycin D and RNA injections enhanced learning, while puromycin was without effect. The authors interpreted these results to indicate that the RNA injection or the inhibition of the normal RNA synthesis by actinomycin D caused an increased availability of nucleotides for new syntheses. Puromycin, cycloheximide, and actinomycin D reversibly inhibited the olfactory bulbar discrimination between home water and other natural waters in the homing salmon (Oshima et al., 1969).

An important study in this respect is that by Laudien (1975). He trained goldfish to take food from cups of different colors on the next day after the intracranial injection of any of a number of known inhibitors of the protein synthesis (puromycin, cycloheximide, 6-azauridine, actinomycin C, and others). Although these drugs affected the frequency of choice between the cups and thus probably the activity of the fishes, none of them affected the acquired color discrimination in tests performed on days 1 and 3 after training (Laudien, 1975, 1977b).

The study of Laudien (1975) appears to indicate that learning instigated by positive reinforcement is not inhibited by inhibitors by protein synthesis. This important result would be more convincing if the inhibitors of protein synthesis had been applied at a time more close to that of the actual training.

As the time of the application of puromycin is critical for its effect on the retention of avoidance learning (Agranoff et al., 1965), it may also be so in positively reinforced conditioning. Ohi (1977) injected actinomycin D intracranially into goldfish 3–4 hours before the first training session for a positively reinforced discrimination learning task. During the successive 4 days of the experiment, the retention from a day to the next ('long term memory') was impaired, while there was no effect on the retention acquired and tested within the same day ('short term memory').

Magnesium pemoline has been reported to facilitate the synthesis of RNA and is therefore suggested to increase the rate of acquisition and to prolong retention. Olson et al. (1973) studied the habituation of a simple innate response in goldfish. In a tall, narrow tank the fish typically swim up and down at a fairly constant rate. A buzzer stimulus given during the ascent inhibits the upward swimming so that the fish will now remain close to the bottom of the tank. When the stimulus is repeated, this response habituates, i.e., the fish gradually resume the original latency of upward swimming. An intraperitoneal injection of magnesium pemoline greatly increased the ascending latencies for the first trials with buzzer stimulus without affecting the spontaneous activity. This may be interpreted as sensitization to the stimulus. Gonzalez and Elder (1972) earlier reported that magnesium pemoline decreases the spontaneous activity of goldfish; this discrepancy may depend on the experimental conditions.

It is not easy to interpret the results of the studies of inhibitors of protein or RNA synthesis on learning and memory in fish. One of the ideas beyond these studies is that the learning of any performance entails either: (a) the synthesis of a memory-specific protein sequence by some cells of the brain; or (b) the synthesis of proteins necessary for an alteration of the synaptic transmission, or for the growth of synaptic connections between some cells of the brain (Agranoff and Klinger, 1964; Agranoff et al., 1964). Another inherent assumption is that an inhibition on the general protein synthesis to 60 to 95 percent is sufficient to block or impair the synthesis of the relevant proteins.

It is unfortunate that most of the pertinent studies have been based on the learning paradigm of avoidance conditioning. Those few in which a positive reinforcement has been used (Batkin et al., 1966; Laudien, 1975) have shown that the inhibitors of protein synthesis do not affect such types of learning or memory. What remains to be explained is why the outcome of avoidance conditioning only seems to be affected by these drugs. On the basis of their experiments, Potts and Bitterman (1967) suggested that the inhibition of protein synthesis by puromycin rather interferes with the fixation of conditioned fear than with the fixation of a specific learned performance.

One may speculate that there is a "fear factor," and perhaps also an "antifear factor," both peptides, which are synthetized in the brain. They may be similar to the hypothalamic releasing and inhibiting factors, liberins and statins, or to the "scotophobin"-type of peptides, suggested to occur in mammals by Ungar et al. (1972); or actually identical with one or more of these. The fear factor would affect such autonomic sensations, the central projections of which would mediate experiences of fear and anxiety. In the view of such an hypothesis, it is interesting to see whether anxiolytic drugs affect learning and memory in fish.

### b.  Effects of Ethyl Alcohol

As stated before, fishes are suitable as test animals for the study of behavioral effects of alcohol. Goldfish have been used in studies on the state-dependence of memory, on the development of behavioral tolerance, on the stimulating effect of low concentrations, and on the effect on conflict behavior.

Ryback (1969a, 1969b) trained goldfish in a continuous Y-maze until they showed 18 correct turns out of 20. The fish were trained either in 4 mg/ml ethyl alcohol solution or in water, and were retrained 3 days later at either of these conditions. High retention of maze performance was found in fish trained first in water and then retrained in alcohol, as well as in the groups that were trained and retrained in the same medium—either water or alcohol. Those fish that were initially trained in alcohol showed poor performance when retested in water. This indicates state-dependence of memory. However, if fish that had been trained under alcohol were placed immediately after training into a higher concentration of alcohol, which produces drunken behavior, they did not show retention even when re-trained under the original alcohol level (Ryback, 1969b). Those fish that were exposed to the higher concentration 24 hours after training showed retention in retraining. Thus, if the "blackout" period was induced immediately after training, no memory of the training could be elicited. The fish learned more poorly both a Y-maze and shock-avoidance responses in a solution of bourbon whisky with a high congener content than in a solution with equivalent pure ethyl alcohol concentration (Ryback, 1969c, 1970).

Alcohol (6 and 8.5 mg/ml) seems to facilitate the early stages of learning of dark-avoidance when a light-off signal is paired with an electric shock (Petty et al., 1973). This may be due to the reduction of the stressful effects and anxiety caused by the shocks received by the fish, especially in the early phase of avoidance learning. Also, a pretraining exposure of the fish for 3 to 6 hours to alcohol solution increases their levels of correct responding during the acquisition (Bryant et al., 1973b). When goldfish are trained in a position discrimination task that is then reversed, alcohol (4 mg/ml) apparently facilitates the short-term memory of the information about the reversal (Ryback, 1976). It is therefore possible that alcohol at low concentrations can act as a stimulant of learning.

Studies on the behavioral tolerance of fish to alcohol were also originated by Ryback (1969c). The performance of goldfish in a continuous Y-maze was poor at high alcohol levels, but a stay of 6 hours in the alcohol solution enhanced it to the level of water controls.

Goldfish usually avoid a high-intensity light stimulus. The avoidance responses are initially decreased in an alcohol solution (0.8 percent), but a reversible tolerance develops in about 30 hours through a characteristic biphasic time course of responsiveness (Goodwin et al., 1971). This time course may in part depend on the increased sensitivity to light caused by alcohol.

The motor disturbance appearing as overturn of goldfish may also be used as a criterion in the studies on the development of alcohol tolerance (Greizerstein and Smith, 1973). However, at high concentrations, no tolerance seems to develop in five tests, and the brain alcohol·levels at the overturn are not changed. Therefore, the previous multiple experiences of the overturn test did not as such contribute to the tolerance effect (Greizerstein and Smith, 1974). Neither did the congeners present in bourbon whisky affect the development of tolerance (Greizerstein, 1977).

Hungry goldfish can be trained to press a lever to obtain food. In a study by Geller et al. (1974), the reinforcement schedule was later changed so that food rewards were given only after variable time intervals averaging 2 minutes. A light signal was then introduced to indicate intermittent changes to a continuous reinforcement schedule. At a later stage, a punishment was added so that the fish were both rewarded with a worm and also received an electric shock. Increasing of the intensity of the shock gradually produced the suppression of the lever-pressing. Sodium phenobarbital attenuated this suppression caused by conflict, perhaps by its anxiolytic action, while alcohol was without effect. A similar attenuation of conditioned emotional suppression without sedation was caused by reserpine in the African mouthbreeder fish *Tilapia macrocephala* (Wilson et al., 1970).

### c. Effects of Other Psychoactive Drugs

Most of the studies concerning the effects of drugs on learning and memory in fishes and in other poikilothermic animals have attempted to answer either of two important questions: (1) is an active protein synthesis in the brain necessary for the formation of long-time memory, and (2) what are the mechanisms of alcohol amnesia. However, the various psychopharmaca available can be used as powerful tools in other approaches to the mechanisms of learning and memory; and, on the other hand, the results of learning experiments may give information on the action mechanisms of these drugs.

Rensch and Dücker (1966) trained pond-living goldfish *Carassius auratus gibelio* to discriminate between two optical patterns using food reward. The fish were tested for retention at intervals of 12 days, from the day 12 after the training to the day 108. During half of each interval, the experimental fish were kept in a solution of chlorpromazine (0.125–0.250 $\mu$g/ml), while the controls were kept in water. The fish treated with chlorpromazine during the interval between the training and the tests showed higher retention. It is possible that the tranquilizing effect of chlorpromazine decreased the adverse effect of later interference on established memory.

The spontaneous upstream swimming of goldfish to a quiet water area above the flow inlet will be suppressed by a single electric shock received in the quiet water. A treatment of the fish with the volatile convulsion-inducing drug flurothyl for 16 minutes after the training, enhanced the retention of the avoidance behavior, as measured by the latency to enter the quiet water area in experiments performed 16, 64, and 256 hours later (Riege and Cherkin, 1973). This retroactive facilitation of learned avoidance by flurothyl was found whether the fish were trained and treated at 25, 20, or 15 C. Flurothyl treatment did not affect the retention in non-contingently shocked control fish.

Flurothyl also causes neuromotor disturbances in the rainbow trout *Salmo gairdneri*, and one of the results of such disturbance is the overturn of the fishes. The latency of overturn in flurothyl solutions depends on the concentration and temperature (Riege and Cherkin, 1976). The retention of the suppression of spontaneous upstream swimming caused by a single electric shock was tested one day after the training. Low concentrations of flurothyl enhanced the retention, and high concentrations impaired it, regardless of the occurrence of convulsions during the treatment (Riege and Cherkin, 1976).

Piracetam (2-oxo-1-pyrrolidone acetamide), a compound chemically related to GABA, has been in experimental use as a drug facilitating learning and memory. Goldfish immersed in a solution of piracetam showed better performance in avoidance conditioning to a light-off stimulus paired with an electric shock during the fourth and fifth days of the training (Bryant et al., 1973a). In addition, a pretraining exposure of 2 days to piracetam resulted in a more rapid acquisition of the avoidance task. These results could not be explained as changes in the general activity level.

Another explanation seems to emerge from a study with the anticonvulsive compound n-dipropylacetate (DPA), which increases the concentration of GABA in the brain. Misslin et al. (1976) studied the effects of this drug on the acquisition of an avoidance response in goldfish. DPA was administered in water 45 minutes before each training session given on 3 successive days. DPA at the lowest concentration used (3 μg/ml) increased the frequency of conditioned avoidance responses during the first day. Higher concentrations (15 and 30 μg/ml) decreased the performance on the second and third day. The authors interpret the increased acquisition caused by the low dose level as an outcome of the anxiolytic action on the drug.

It is interesting from the standpoint of the hypothesis of a consolidation phase in the formation of memory, that the effects of stimulants and sedatives on retention may also depend on the time of their application. Liu and Braud (1974) found that the stimulant picrotoxin injected intracranially in goldfish 5 minutes before, immediately, and 1 hour after the first training session facilitated avoidance performance in subsequent training sessions. Pentobarbital injected before or immediately after training impaired later performance. Picrotoxin injected 4 hours after training was without effect, as was pentobarbital injected 0.5 or 1 hour after training. The drugs were used at concentrations that apparently did not affect the general activity of the fish.

When goldfish are immersed for 24 hours in water containing the MAO inhibitor pargyline, the brain concentrations of NA and DA are increased (Stahl et al., 1971). L-DOPA causes an increase in NA concentration, but a slight decrease in DA concentration. On the day after the exposure of fish to L-DOPA, the rate of acquisition of an avoidance task was enhanced by 92 percent, but depressed on the second day. Pargyline decreased the acquisition on the second and third day after treatment. The increased brain DA level seems thus to be related with enhanced learning.

Sahagian and Ingle (1977) trained goldfish in a continuous Y-maze. A pretreatment for 30 minutes in water containing 1.25 μg/ml d-amphetamine increased the rate of learning while 2 μg/ml was without effect.

The effects of psychopharmaca on performance in learning experiments may also be affected by the reinforcement schedule. Reserpine (4 mg/kg) injected intramuscularly inhibited responding during extinction in African mouthbreeder fish *Tilapia macrocephala* conditioned with consistent reinforcement, but not in fish conditioned with partial reinforcement (Haralson and Clement, 1968).

These results support the view that modifications of the catecholamine levels in the brain affect different types of learning in fishes. The cholinergic system is, of course, also involved. When injected subcutaneously, the cholinesterase inhibitor armin (o-ethyl-o-(4-nitrophenyl)-ethyl phosphonate reduced the brain cholinesterase activity to 80 percent of the control levels in the fish *Serranus scriba* (Rosič et al., 1974). The same dose of armin depressed avoidance conditioning with a similar time course of the effect. No other disturbances of behavior were observed with this dose level.

It is difficult to summarize this variety of studies in which different types of psychopharmaca have been used in connection with different learning paradigms. In a positive reinforcement situation, long-time treatment with a tranquilizer seems to enhance retention, either by decreasing the interference caused by later learning and activity on established memory, or by diminishing the effects of secondary situation-dependent factors on performance. The retention of a single-shock conditioned avoidance response can be increased by a treatment with low concentration of a convulsant after training. On the other hand, the rate of acquisition of avoidance responses conditioned by multiple shocks seems to be enhanced by increased GABA or DA concentrations in the brain. These effects are perhaps related to the fear-reducing, respectively activity-increasing effects of these neurotransmitters.

## 3.  Learning and Memory in Other Poikilotherms

Remarkably, the effects of psychoactive drugs on the learning and memory have been seldom studied in other poikilothermic animals, except insects and fishes. Habituation consists of the waning of a response to a repeatedly presented stimulus, and is often regarded as a simple form of learning. It has been shown to occur in all animals, including the aneural protozoans. Gardner and Applewhite (1970) studied the effects of a number of protein and RNA synthesis inhibitors on habituation of the ciliate protozoan *Spirostomum ambiguum* to mechanical shocks. Inhibition of protein synthesis up to 95 percent had no effect on habituation, and RNA inhibition up to 89 percent by 5-fluorouracil had only a slight effect. Apparently, no very active protein and RNA synthesis is necessary for habituation.

Another instance of habituation is the waning of the shadow reflex in the barnacles *Balanus*. The rhythmic beating of the cirral legs of these sessile crustaceans is interrupted by a sudden decrease in light intensity, which also causes the closure of their shell. Repeated short decreases of light intensity cause the habituation of this response. Waldes (1938) showed that externally applied ACh and atropine strongly affected the shadow reflex. In later experiments, ACh decreased the retention of habituation, i.e., enhanced the recovery of the response (Lagerspetz and Kivivuori, 1970). This result is in agreement with the hypothesis that habituation is caused by depletion of the neurotransmitter in question.

The structurally and functionally well-known nervous system of the marine snail *Aplysia californica* has long been a favorite study object in the cellular neurophysiology of behavior (for an excellent review, see Kandel, 1976). Several phenomena of nervous and behavioral plasticity in *Aplysia* have been thoroughly analyzed by neurophysiological methods and furnish suitable model systems for neuropsychopharmacological work. The rate of habituation of the gill withdrawal reflex (Peretz et al., 1971) and the siphon withdrawal reflex (Newby, 1973) are increased by ACh and the cholinesterase inhibitor physostigmine. Inhibitory ACh neurons seem to affect these reflexes. High concentrations of DA block the habituation of the siphon withdrawal reflex (Newby, 1973). Also, this result is in agreement with the hypothesis that habituation in single junctions is caused by reduction of the presynaptically released neurotransmitter.

Frogs do rapid prey-catching movements towards a moving worm-like object. If these are restricted and do not lead to rewarding consummatory behavior, the frequency of responses is soon reduced. Ingle (1973) found that in two experimental situations, ethyl alcohol decreased the rate of habituation. It is possible that alcohol induced a disinhibition within the visuomotor mechanism of the frog. This test could perhaps be useful in studies on the effects of psychoactive drugs on disinhibitory processes.

## G.  PERSPECTIVES FOR COMPARATIVE PSYCHOPHARMACOLOGY

### 1.  Conclusions

The bulk of the more than 1.1 million extant animal species are poikilothermic, i.e., do not possess the physiological mechanisms of thermoregulation typical for mammals and birds. Since the introduction of psychopharmaca in the early 1950s, their effects on the behavior of poikilothermic animals have been studied, first occasionally, and later with growing interest.

Neurochemical studies have shown the almost ubiquitous occurrence of many neurotransmitter substances. The similarities found on the molecular level and in part on the cellular level in different animals are in contrast with the large variation in the structures of their nervous systems and in their behavior. Especially on the behavioral level, which reflects the interactions of the organism and its environment, the scientist is confronted with important phenomena that cannot be reduced to simple physiological or behavioral functions. In the interpretation of these phenomena, the previously stored information and its effects on the handling of new information must be taken into account.

It is important to be aware of the dangers of reductionism, but it is equally important to notice the complexity of the central mechanisms that determine even the behavior of many poikilothermic animals. Therefore, students of comparative psychopharmacology have been forced to ascribe such properties as fear, anxiety, and attentiveness even to lower animals. This has been especially typical for research on the learning and memory, which belong to the so-called higher functions of the nervous systems.

Of the simpler types of behavior, relatively much attention has been paid to the pharmacology of spontaneous motor activity. Although 5-HT increases cell motility and also the spontaneous motor activity of arthropods and mollusks, its effect on the motor activity of vertebrates is opposite. The sedative action of reserpine in the frog can be potentiated by tricyclic antidepressants, which also induce muscle twitches. A screening test for tymoleptic drugs is based on these observations (Lapin et al., 1970). The frequency of web-building in spiders and the geometrical structure of orb-webs are affected by a number of psychoactive drugs, which suggests the use of the web-building in spiders as a general screening test for different psychopharmaca (Witt, 1956).

The intraspecific and interspecific aggression of some poikilothermic animals is another type of complicated stereotypic behavior. Studies on the aggressive behavior of ants suggest that monoaminergic neurons of the central nervous system are involved in its mediation in these insects (Tarchalska et al., 1975; Kostowski et al., 1975a), as they are in mammals and also possibly in fishes (Baenninger, 1968).

The usefulness of fishes as experimental animals in psychophysiological and psychopharmacological work has been pointed out by several authors (Cutting et al., 1959; Ingle, 1965; Braud, 1970; Ryback, 1970). The effects of different types of psychopharmaca on the aggressive behavior of the Siamese fighting fish and the convict cichlid have been studied. These experiments show, e.g., that the predatory and sexual arousal are mediated by different mechanisms than the intraspecific aggression (Avis and Peeke, 1975; Figler, 1973; Figler et al., 1975). On the other hand, they show that the observation of a single behavior pattern like aggressive display is often not enough to discriminate between the effects of different types of psychopharmaca. It is interesting that fighting fish can learn to associate neutral stimuli with pharmacologically affected state of aggression (Braud and Weibel, 1969).

Fishes, especially goldfish, have been extensively used in studies on the psychopharmacology of learning and memory. The effectiveness of drugs depends, among other factors, on the relation of the time of application to the time of training. In avoidance-conditioning experiments, the inhibition of protein synthesis seems to impair the later performance in retention tests. Several mechanisms of this effect have been suggested: (1) the impairment of specific memory fixation through interference with the synthesis of memory-specific proteins, or (2) through inhibition of the synthesis of proteins necessary for synaptic changes or synaptic growth (Agranoff and Klinger, 1964); (3) impairment of the fixation of learned fear through the same mechanisms (Potts and Bitterman, 1967); (4) the inhibition of the synthesis of a peptide factor mediating the effects of fear. The results of the few experiments with positive reinforcement do not speak for the importance of unaffected protein synthesis for memory fixation.

In experiments with ethyl alcohol, goldfish show state-dependent learning and induced tolerance to the effects of alcohol. The effects of other psychoactive substances have also been studied in fishes, mainly using the conditioned-avoidance technique. This learning paradigm has also been used with insect preparations to study the effects of inhibitors of protein synthesis and the roles of neurotransmitters. The few experiments with other poikilothermic animals have been mainly concerned with the effects of neurotransmitters and drugs on the habituation of simple reflexes.

## 2. Suggestions for Further Research

In spite of the dangers of reductive explanations of human behavior and the difficulties in the comparisons of the results of clinical studies with those of the work on animal models, comparative psychopharmacology is a field very much alive today. There are many areas of study in which the choice of poikilothermic animals for test objects would obviously further the biomedical research on psychoactive drugs. Some of them are mentioned below.

### a. Temperature Effects

The effects of psychoactive drugs in small laboratory mammals are often obscured by the lack of monitoring and control of the body temperature. These animals have a very labile thermoregulation, which is affected by a variety of drugs. The side effect of the drug on body temperature may mask, reverse, or exaggerate the actual effects to be studied.

One of the advantages of the use of poikilothermic animals in psychopharmacological research is that they can be studied at different body temperatures and nevertheless be considered as "normal." This makes it possible to study the interactions of the effects of drugs and temperature, which are largely unexplored (see however, Cano Puerta, 1959; Cherkin and Catchpool, 1964; Neale et al., 1973b; Riege and Cherkin, 1976). Such studies could elucidate the action mechanisms of psychoactive drugs, especially as temperature has definite effects on the release and metabolism of neurotransmitters in poikilothermic animals (Brodie et al., 1964; Mirolli and Welsh, 1964; Harri, 1972a, 1972b; Stefano and Catapane, 1977).

### b. Behavioral Selection of Temperature

Another interesting aspect is the temperature-preference behavior, shown by all animals so far studied, even by protozoans. All animals, when placed in a temperature gradient, seem to prefer a certain range of temperature. This preferred temperature depends on the species, on the thermal history of the test animals, and on a number of other conditions. Also, drugs affect it. Sodium pentobarbital decreases the selected mean temperature in the Atlantic salmon *Salmo salar* and in the guppy *Poecilia reticulata*, and increases it in the rainbow trout *Salmo gairdneri* (Ogilvie and Fryer, 1971; Fryer and Ogilvie, 1974). It is also known, that an injection of bacteria increases the selected temperature in fishes, frogs, and lizards, while the antipyretic drug acetaminophen counteracts this effect (Reynolds and Covert, 1977). Temperature-selection experiments may be combined with operant conditioning, since goldfish can be trained to control the water temperature by lever-pressing (Rozin, 1968). Studies with psychoactive drugs could not only elucidate the mechanisms of the behavioral responses to external temperatures, but they could also be useful in the development of screening tests for drugs.

### c. Induced Tolerance and Drug Metabolism

Repeated administration of a psychoactive drug often induces tolerance to its effects. Poikilothermic animals have not very often been used in studies on the development and mechanisms of induced tolerance to other psychoactive substances, except ethyl alcohol (Ryback, 1969c; Goodwin et al., 1971; Greizerstein and Smith, 1973, 1974; Greizerstein, 1977). As the nervous systems of animals show a large structural variation, it is possible that a comparative approach to these problems would be rewarding.

Tolerance develops to the depressing effect of $\Delta^9$-tetrahydro-cannabinol on aggressive behavior of Siamese fighting fish (González, 1971). This hallucinogen also inhibits the righting reflex in the frog. Complete tolerance to this effect is found after 3 doses injected every other day (Abel, 1963).

In spite of their importance, remarkably little work has been done on the effects of opiates. Josefsson and Johansson (1979) have studied the inhibitory effect of opiates on pinocytosis in the protozoan *Amoeba proteus*. Tolerance to this effect develops already within a few hours (Johansson and Josefsson, 1979).

In the early 1960's, most studies on the metabolism of xenobiotic compounds in poikilothermic animals failed to show any active biotransformation, partly because the used assay temperature (37 C) was too high for many enzymes of poikilotherms (Adamson, 1967). There are still almost no studies on the metabolism of psychoactive drugs in poikilotherms.

### d. Learning and Memory with Positive Reinforcement

The biochemical mechanisms of learning and memory have been the subject of a number of studies, especially on fish. However, very little attention has been paid to the use of positive reinforcement as compared with avoidance learning with electric shocks as punishment. The study of Laudien (1975) on the effects of inhibitors of protein and RNA syntheses on retention in goldfish is exceptional in this respect, and such approach should be pursued further. There is a lack of systematic studies in which the effects of psychoactive drugs would have been tested using different paradigms of learning. Also, the effects of long-term treatments with psychopharmaca have been studied in very few cases (Rensch and Dücker, 1966). Studies on structurally and functionally well-defined nervous systems, like that of *Aplysia* (Kandel, 1976), will probably yield valuable information in the future on the effects of psychopharmaca on learning and memory.

### e. Responses to Noxious Stimuli and Chemical Compounds

The nociceptive threshold has been studied in frogs using the hot-plate technique (Nistri and Pepeu, 1974). While both morphine and oxotremorine increase the brain level of ACh in frogs, only the latter drug has an analgesic effect in these animals. Very little is know about the central mechanisms of analgesia in poikilothermic animals.

Organisms from aneural (Koshland, 1974; Hauser et al., 1975) to higher animals respond behaviorally to various chemical compounds. Substances eliciting feeding responses have been studied even in such relatively simple animals as the coelenterate *Hydra* (Lenhoff, 1968, 1969) and the planarian *Dugesia dorotocephala* (Ash et al., 1973). Certain aspects of chemotactic behavior have been studied in nematodes (Dusenbery, 1976), in which the neuroanatomy is known in detail and which are also otherwise suitable for neurogenetical studies. The possible effects of psychopharmaca on chemotactic behavior is a virtually unexplored field.

### f. Side Effects

In view of the variety of nervous system in animals, it is possible that some of the side effects of psychopharmaca in mammals would be more easily accessible for experimentation in poikilothermic animals. Such work should proceed in a close contact with studies on laboratory mammals and with clinical experiences.

### g. Action Mechanisms and Specific Screening Tests

The use of frogs for the study of 5-HT mediated central processes is advantageous because of the minimal interference caused by adrenergic mechanisms. The test devised by Lapin et al. (1970) for the screening of tymoleptic drugs is based on this special characteristic of the central nervous system of the frog. There may also be other types of behavior that mainly depend on the function of a single neurotransmitter in poikilothermic animals. These could be useful in the study of the action mechanisms of psychopharmaca as well as in the development of specific screening tests.

## H. SUMMARY

Studies of the effects of psychoactive drugs and neurotransmitters on the behavior of invertebrates and poikilothermic vertebrates are reviewed.

Dangers òf reductive explanations are pointed out. Results and suggestions are given concerning the use of poikilothermic animals (1) in the development of screening tests, (2) in experiments on the action mechanisms of psychopharmaca, and (3) in the use of psychoactive drugs in the study of the mechanisms of animal behavior.

## ACKNOWLEDGEMENTS

The author is grateful to Mrs. Svea Söderström for competent secretarial help and to the Academy of Finland for financial support.

## I.  REFERENCES

Abel, E.L. (1973). Development of tolerance to Δ⁹-THC in the frog. *Experientia* 29:1527–1528.

Abramson, H.A. (1957). Blocking of the LSD-25 reaction in Siamese fighting fish, in *Neuropharmacology*. Third Conference 1956, H.A. Abramson, ed. Macy Foundation, New York. pp. 9–27.

Abramson, H.A., and Evans, T.L. (1954). Lysergic acid diethylamide (LSD-25). II. Psychobiological effects on the Siamese fighting fish. *Sci.* 120:990–991.

Abramson, H.A., and Jarvik, M.E. (1955). Lysergic acid diethvlamide (LSD-25): Effects on snails. *J. Psychol.* 40:337–340.

Adamson, R.H. (1963). Drug metabolism in marine vertebrates. *Fed. Proc.* 26:1047–1055.

Agranoff, B.W., and Davis, R.E. (1968). The use of fishes in studies on memory formation, in *The Central Nervous System and Fish Behavior* D. Ingle, ed. Univ. of Chicago Press, Chicago. pp. 193–201.

Agranoff, B.W., and Klinger, P.D. (1964). Puromycin effect on memory fixation in the goldfish. *Sci.* 146:952–953.

Agranoff, B.W., Davis, R.E., and Brink, J.J. (1966). Chemical studies on memory fixation in goldfish. *Brain Res.* 1:303–309.

Agranoff, B.W., Davis, R.E., and Brink, J.J. (1965). Memory fixation in the goldfish. *Proc. Nat. Acad. Sci.* 54:788–793.

Agranoff, B.W., Davis, R.E., Casola, L., and Lim, R. (1967). Actinomycin D blocks formation of memory of shock-avoidance in goldfish. *Sci.* 158:1600–1601.

Applewhite, P.B. (1972). Drugs affecting sensitivity to stimuli in the plant *Mimosa* and the protozoan *Spirostomum*. *Physiol. Behav.* 9:869–871.

Ash, J.F., McClure, W.O., and Hirsch, J. (1973). Chemical studies of a factor which elicits feeding behavior in *Dugesia dorotocephala*. *Anim. Behav.* 21:796–800.

Atherton, R.W. (1975). Neurochemical effects on sperm cell motility in *Strongylocentrotus purpuratus*, the purple sea urchin. *Comp. Biochem. Physiol.* 50C:21–26.

Avis, H.H., and Peeke. H.Y.S. (1975). Differentiation by morphine òf two types of aggressive behavior in the convict cichlid (*Cichlasoma nigrofasciatum*). *Psychopharmacologia* 43:287–288.

Bacq, Z.M. (1947). L'acétylcholine et l'adrénaline chez les Invertebrés. *Biolog. Rev.* 22:73–91.

Baenninger, R. (1968). Catecholamines and social relations in Siamese fighting fish. *Anim. Behav.* 16:442–447.

Baslow, M.H. (1969). *Marine Pharmacology*. Williams & Wilkins, Baltimore XIV:286.

Batkin, S., Woodard, W.T., Cole, R.E., and Hall, J.B. (1966). RNA and actinomycin-D enhancement of learning in the carp. *Psychonom. Sci.* 5:345–346.

Boissier, J., and Pagny, J. (1959). L'utilisation du poisson combattant du Siam (*Betta splendens*, Regan) pour l'étude des psycholeptiques. *Thér.* 14:324–331.

Braud, W.G. (1970). The goldfish as a subject for psychological and physiological research. *J. Biolog. Psychol.* 12:61–64.

Braud, W.G., and Broussard, W.J. (1973). Effects of puromycin on memory for shuttlebox extinction in goldfish and barpress extinction in rats. *Pharmacol. Biochem. Behav.* 1:651–656.

Braud, W.G., and Weibel, J.E. (1969). Acquired stimulus control of drug-induced changes in aggressive display in *Betta splendens*. *J. Exper. Anal. Behav.* 12:773–777.

Brodie, B.B., and Bogdanski, D.F. (1964). Biogenic amines and drug action in the nervous system of various vertebrate classes. *Prog. in Brain Res.* 9:234–242.

Brodie, B.B., Bogdanski, D.F., and Bonomi, L. (1964). Formation, storage, and metabolism of serotonin (5-hydroxytryptamine) and catecholamines in lower vertebrates, in *Comparative Neurochemistry* D. Richter, ed. Pergamon Press, Oxford. pp. 367–377.

Brown B.M., and Noble, E.P. (1968). Cycloheximide, amino acid incorporation, and learning in the isolated cockroach ganglion. *Biochem. Pharmacol.* 17:2371–2374.

Brown, B.M., and Noble, E.P. (1967). Cycloheximide and learning in the isolated cockroach ganglion. *Brain Res.* 6:363–366.

Bryant, R.C., Petty, F., and Byrne, W.F. (1973a). Effects of piracetam (SKF 38462) on acquisition, retention, and activity in the goldfish. *Psychopharmacologia* 29:121–130.

Bryant, R.G., Petty, F., Warren, J.L., and Byrne, W.L. (1973b). Facilitation by alcohol of active avoidance acquisition performance in the goldfish. *Pharmacol. Biochem. Behav.* 1:523–529.

Cano Puerta, G. (1959). The effects of tranquilizing drugs on tropical fish. *Arch. Int. Pharmacodyn. Thér.* 121:404–414.

Casola, L., Lim, R., Davis, R.E., and Agranoff, B.W. (1968). Behavioral and biochemical effects of intracranial injection of cytosine arabinoside in goldfish. *Proc. Nat. Acad. Sci.* Washington, D.C. 60:1389–1395.

Cherkin, A., and Catchpool, J.F. (1964). Temperature dependence of anesthesia in goldfish. *Sci.* 144:1460–1462.

Christiansen, A., Baum, R., and Witt, P.N. (1962). Changes in spider webs brought about by mescaline, psilocybin, and an increase in body weight. *J. Pharmacol.* 136:31–37.

Cooper, P.D., Umemoto, L., Friend, W.G., and Hartwick, W.B. (1971). Effects of drugs on the behaviour of the Carpenter Ant, *Camponotus herculeanus*. Comp. Gen. Pharmacol. 2:120–124.

Cottrell, G.A., and Laverack, M.S. (1968). Invertebrate pharmacology. *Ann. Rev. Pharmacol.* 7:273–298.

Crescitelli, F., and Geissman, T.A. (1962). Invertebrate pharmacology: Selected topics. *Ann. Rev. Pharmacol.* 2:143–192.

Cutting, W., Baslow, M., Read, D., and Furst, A. (1959). The use of fish in the evaluation of drugs affecting the central nervous system. *J. Clin. Exper. Psychopathol.* 20:26–32.

Cymborowski, B. (1970). The assumed participation of 5-hydroxytryptamine in regulation of the circadian rhythm of locomotor activity in *Acheta domesticus* L. *Comp. Gen. Pharmacol.* 1:316–322.

Davis, R.E., and Agranoff, B.W. (1966). Stages of memory formation in goldfish: Evidence for an environmental trigger. *Proc. Nat. Acad. Sci.* 55:555–559.

Davis, R.E., Bright, P.J., and Agranoff, B.W. (1965). Effect of ECS and puromycin on memory in fish. *J. Comp. Physiolog. Psychol.* 60:162–166.

Dolce, G., and Garello, L. (1956). La catalessia da serotonina nella *Rana esculenta*: Tecnica sperimentale. *Boll. Soc. Ital. Biol. Sper.* 32:441–443.

Doshi, E., and Huggins, S.E. (1977). Drug-induced brain monoamine depletion and its behavioral correlates in *Caiman sclerops*. *Comp. Biochem. Physio.* 57C:153–157.

Duncan, C.J. (1967). *The Molecular Properties and Evolution of Excitable Cells.* Pergamon Press, Oxford.

Dusenbery, D.B. (1976). Attraction of the nematode *Caenorhabditis elegans* to pyridine. *Comp. Biochem. Physiol.* 53C:1–2.

Eckert, R. (1972). Bioelectric control of ciliary activity. *Sci.* 176:473–481.

isenstein, E.M. (1968). Assessing the influence of pharmacological agents on shock avoidance in simpler systems. *Brain Res.* 11:471–480.

Eisenstein, E.M. (1965). Effects of strychnine sulfate and sodium pentabarbital on shock-avoidance learning in an isolated insect ganglion. Proceedings of 73rd Annual Meeting of the American Psychological Association. 127–128.

Eisenstein, E.M., and Cohen, M.J. (1965). Learning in an isolated prothoracic insect ganglion. *Anim. Behav.* 13:104–108.

Evans, L.T., Abramson, H.A., and Fremont-Smith, N. (1958). Lysergic acid diethylamide (LSD-25): XXVI. Effect on social order of the fighting fish, *Betta splendens. J. Psychol.* 45:263–273.

Evans, L.T., Geronimus, L.H., Kornestsky, C., and Abramson, H.A. (1956). Effect of ergot drugs on *Betta splendens. Sci.* 123:26.

Fänge, R. (1962). Pharmacology of poikilothermic vertebrates and invertebrates. *Pharmacolog. Rev.* 14:281–316.

*Federation Proceedings.* (1967). Proceedings of an International Symposium of Comparative Pharmacology. 26:963–1265.

Figler, M.H. (1973). The effects of chlordiazepoxide (Librium) on the intensity and habituation of agonistic behavior in male Siamese fighting fish. *Psychopharmacologia.* 33:277–292.

Figler, M.H., and Bennett, R.W. (1974). Secobarbital sodium (Seconal) attenuates attack behavior in male Siamese fighting fish. *Fed. Proc.* 33:466.

Figler, M.H., Klein, R.M., and Thompson, C.S. (1975). Chlordiazepoxide (Librium)-induced changes in intraspecific attack and selected non-agonistic behaviors in male Siamese fighting fish. *Psychopharmacologia.* 42:139–145.

Fingerman, S.W. (1976). Circadian rhythms of brain 5-hydroxytryptamine and swimming activity in the teleost, *Fundulus grandis. Comp. Biochem. Physiol.* 54C:49–53.

Florey, E. (1965). Comparative pharmacology: Neurotropic and myotropic compounds. *Ann. Rev. Pharmacol* 5:357–382.

Florey, E. (1961). Comparative physiology: Transmitter substances. *Ann. Rev. Physiol.* 23: 501–528.

Fryer, J.N., and Ogilvie, D.M. (1974). Temperature selection response of Atlantic salmon, *Salmo salar,* and rainbow trout, *Salmo gairdneri,* after exposure to pentobarbital. *Comp. Gen. Pharmacol.* 5:111–116.

Gardner, F.T., and Applewhite, P.B. (1970). Protein and RNA inhibitors and protozoan habituation. *Psychopharmacologia.* 16:430–433.

Geiger, R.S. (1963). The behavior of adult mammalian brain cells in culture. *Int. Rev. Neurobiol.* 5:1–52.

Geller, I., Croy, D.J., and Ryback, R.S. (1974). Effects of ethanol and sodium phenobarbital on conflict behavior of goldfish (*Carassius auratus*). *Pharmacol. Biochem. Behav.* 2:545–548.

Gerschenfeld, H.M. (1973). Chemical transmission in invertebrate central nervous systems and neuromuscular junctions. *Physiolog. Rev.* 53:1–119.

Gerschenfeld, H.M. (1965). Chemical transmitters in invertebrate nervous system. *Symp. Soc. Exper. Biol.* 20:299–323.

Glassman, E., Henderson, A., Cordle, M., Moon, H.M., and Wilson, J.E. (1970). Effect of cycloheximide and actinomycin D on the behaviour of the headless cockroach. *Nat.* 225:967–968.

Gonzalez, L.P., and Elder, S.T. (1972). Depression of spontaneous activity in goldfish by magnesium pemoline. *Psychonom. Sci.* 28:293–294.

González, S.C., Matsudo, V.K.R., and Carlini, E.A. (1971). Effects of marihuana compounds on the fighting behavior of Siamese fighting fish. *Pharmacol.* 6:186–190.

Goodwin, D.W., Dowd, C.P., and Guze, S.B. (1971). Biphasic and reversible adaptation of goldfish to alcohol. *Nat.* 232:654–655.

Goyffon, M., Richard, M., and Vernet, R. (1974). Activité électrique cérébrale spontanée et comportement moteur du Scorpion. Intérêt pharmacologique. *Compt. Rend. Séances Sociét Biol.* 168:1239–1244.

Greizerstein, H.B. (1977). Tolerance to ethanol: Effect of congeners present in bourbon. *Psychopharmacol.* 53:201–203.

Greizerstein, H.B., and Smith, C.M. (1974). Ethanol in goldfish: Effect of prior exposure in a test procedure. *Psychopharmacologia.* 38:345–349.

Greizerstein, H.B., and Smith, C.M. (1973). Development and loss of tolerance to ethanol in goldfish. *J. Pharmacol. Exper. Therapeut.* 187:391–399.

Groh, G., and Lemieuz, M. (1968). The effect of LSD-25 on spider web formation. *Int. J. Addict.* 30:41–53.

Gustafson, T., and Toneby, M. (1970). On the role of serotonin and acetylcholine in sea urchin morphonogenesis. *Exper. Cell Res.* 62:102–117.

Gustafson, T., Lundgren, B., and Treufeldt, R. (1972). Serotonin and contractile activity in the echinopluteus. A study of the cellular basis of larval behaviour. *Exper. Cell Res.* 72:115–139.

Haralson, J.V., and Clement, J.J. (1968). Reserpine and the partial reinforcement effect in the fish *Tilapia H. macrocephala. Psycholog. Rep.* 22:1057–1064.

Harri, M.N.E. (1974). The dependence of imipramine-induced sedation upon central 5-hydroxytryptamine-like activity in the frog. *J. Pharm. Pharmacol.* 26:73–74.

Harri, M.N.E. (1972a). Effect of season and temperature acclimation on the 5-hydroxytryptamine level and utilization in the brain and intestine of the frog, *Rana temporaria. Comp. Gen. Pharmacol.* 3:11–18.

Harri, M.N.E. (1972b). Effect of season and temperature acclimation on the tissue catecholamine level and utilization in the frog, *Rana temporaria. Comp. Gen. Pharmacol.* 3:101–112.

Hauser, D.C.R., Levandowsky, M., and Glassgold, J.M. (1975). Ultrasensitive chemosensory responses by a protozoan to epinephrine and other neurochemicals. *Sci.* 190:285–286.

Hiripi, L., and Salánki, J. (1973). Role of monoamines in the central regulation of periodic activity in *Anodonta cygnea* L. (Pelecypoda), in *Neurobiology of Invertebrates.* J. Salánki, ed. Akadémiai Kiadó, Budapest. pp. 391–401.

Horner, J.C., Longo, N., and Bitterman, M.E. (1961). A shuttle box for fish and control circuit of general applicability. *Am. J. Psychol.* 74:114–120.

Horridge, G.A. (1962). Learning of log position by the ventral nerve cord in headless insects. *Proc. Roy. Soc. London* B 157:33–52.

Houston, A.H., and Woods, R.J. (1976). Influence of temperature upon tricaine methane sulphonate uptake and induction of anesthesia in rainbow trout (*Salmo gairdneri*). *Comp. Biochem. Physiol.* 54C:1–6.

Hunn, J.B., and Allen, J.L. (1974). Movement of drugs across the gills of fishes. *Ann. Rev. Pharmacol.* 14:47–55.

Huot, L., Corrivault, G.W., and Bourbeau, G. (1960). Less substances neuroleptiques et le comportement des insectes. I. L'influence de la reserpine sur la ponte de *Tribolium confusum.* Duval. *Arch. Int. Physiol.* 68:577–585.

Ingle, D.J. (1965). The use of the fish in neuropsychology. *Perspect. Biol. Med.* 8:241–260.

Ingle, D. (1973). Reduction of habituation of prey-catching activity by alcohol intoxication in the frog. *Behav. Biol.* 8:123–129.

Jarvik, M.E. (1957). Effect of LSD-25 on snails, in *Neuropharmacology.* Third Conference 1956, H.A. Abramson, ed. Macy Foundation, New York. pp. 29–38.

Johansson, P., and Josefsson, J.-O. (1979). Rapid development of tolerance to opiates in *Amoeba proteus*. *Acta Physiol. Scand. Suppl.* 473:67.

Johnson, F.N. (1979): Lithium effects on social aggregation in the goldfish (*Carassius auratus*). *Medical Biology* 57:102-106.

Josefsson, J.-O., and Johansson, P. (1979). Naloxone-reversible effect of opioids on pinocytosis in *Amoeba proteus. Nature* 282:78-80.

Juorio, A.V. (1973). The distribution of catecholamines in the hypothalamus and other brain areas of some lower vertebrates. *J. Neurochem.* 20:641-645.

Kandel, E.R. (1976). *Cellular Basis of Behavior*. Freeman, San Fransisco.

Katona, F., and Wollemann, M. (1964). The effect of phenothiazines on some invertebrate animals. A comparative physiological survey, in *Comparative Neurochemistry*. R. Richter, ed. Pergamon Press, Oxford. pp. 445-450.

Kehoe, J.-S., and Marder, E. (1976). Identification and effects of neural transmitters in invertebrates. *Ann. Rev. Pharmacol. Toxicol.* 16:245-268.

Keller, D.L., and Umbreit, W.W. (1956). Chemically altered "permanent" behaviour patterns in fish and their cure by reserpine. *Sci.* 124:407.

Kerkut, G.A., Oliver, G.W.O., Rick, J.T., and Walker, R.J. (1970). The effects of drugs on learning in a simple preparation. *Comp. Gen. Pharmacol.* 1:437-483.

Koshland, D.E., Jr. (1974). Chemotaxis as a model for sensory systems. *FEBS Letters.* Supp. 40:53-59.

Koshtoyants, Kh. S., Buznikov, G.A., and Manukhin, B.N. (1961). The possible role of 5-hydroxytryptamine in the motor activity of embryos of some marine gastropods. *Comp. Biochem. Physiol.* 3:20-26.

Kostowski, W. (1968). A note on the effects of some cholinergic and anticholinergic drugs on the aggressive behaviour and spontaneous electrical activity of the central nervous system in the ant, *Formica rufa. J. Pharm. Pharmacol.* 20:381-384.

Kostowski, W. (1966). A note on the effects of some psychotropic drugs on the aggressive behaviour in the ant, *Formica rufa. J. Phar. Pharmacol.* 18:747-749.

Kostowski, W., and Tarchalska, B. (1972). The effects of some drugs affecting brain 5-HT on the aggressive behavior and spontaneous electrical activity of the central nervous system of the ant, *Formica rufa. Brain Res.* 38:143-149.

Kostowski, W., Beck, J., and Mészáros, J. (1966). Studies on the effect of certain neurohormones and psychotropic drugs on bioelectric activity of the central nervous system and behavior in ants, *Formica rufa. L. Acta Physiol. Polon.* 17:98-110.

Kostowski, W., Beck, J., and Mészáros, J. (1965). Drugs affecting the behaviour and spontaneous bioelectrical activity of the central nervous system in the ant, *Formica rufa. J. Pharm. Pharmacol.* 17:253-255.

Kostowski, W., Tarchalska-Krynska, B., and Markowska, L. (1975a). Aggressive behavior and brain serotonin and catecholamines in ants, *Formica rufa. Pharmacol. Biochem. Behav.* 3:717-720.

Kostowski, W., Tarchalska, B., and Wanchowicz, B. (1975b). Brain catecholamines, spontaneous bioelectrical activity and aggressive behavior in ants, *Formica rufa. Pharmacol. Biochem. Behav.* 3:337-342.

Krebs, H.A. (1975). The August Kroghs principle: "For many problems there is an animal on which it can be most conveniently studied. *J. Exper. Zool.* 194:221-226.

Lagerspetz, K.M.J. (1964). Studies on the aggressive behaviour of mice. *Ann. Acad. Scientiar. Fennicae.* Series B, 131/3:1-131.

Lagerspetz, K.M.J., and Ekqvist, K. (1978). Failure to induce aggression in inhibited and in genetically non-aggressive mice, through injections of ethyl alcohol. *Agg. Behav.* (In press.)

Lagerspetz, K.M.J., and Hautojärvi, S. (1967). The effect of prior aggressive or sexual arousal on subsequent aggressive or sexual reactions in male mice. *Scand. J. Psychol.* 8:1-6.

Lagerspetz, K.Y.H., and Kivivuori, L. (1970). The rate and retention of the habituation of the shadow reflex in *Balanus improvisus* (Cirripedia). *Anim. Behav.* 18:616–620.

Lapin, I.P., and Oxenkrug, G.F. (1969). Intensification of the central serotonergic processes as a possible determinant of the thymoleptic effect. *Lancet.* 18:132–136.

Lapin, I.P., Osipova, S.V., Uskova, N.V., and Stabrowski, E.M. (1968). Synergism of imipramine and desmethylimipramine with reserpine in the frog. Interaction with 5-hydroxytryptophan and 2-bromolysergic diethylamide (BOL-148). *Arch. Int. Pharmacodyn. Thér.* 174:37–49.

Lapin, I.P., Oxenkrug, G.F., Osipova, S.V., and Uskova, N.V. (1970). The frog as a subject for screening thymoleptic drugs. *J. Pharm. Pharmacol.* 22:781–782.

Laudien, H. (1977a). *Physiologie des Gedächtnisses.* Quelle and Meyer, Heidelberg.

Laudien, H. (1977b): Langzeitgedächtnis und Proteinbiosynthese. Versuche mit Goldfischen (*Carassius auratus auratus* L.). *Zoologischer Anzeiger (Jena)* 199:19–28.

Laudien, H. (1975). Über die Wirkung einiger Inhibitoren der Protein-Biosynthese auf Aktivität und Lernverhalten beim Goldfish (*Carassius auratus auratus* L.) *Zeit. Tierpsychol.* 38:436–443.

Leake, L.D., and Taylor, I.B. (1972). The role of GABA in learning in the cockroach? *Comp. Gen. Pharmacol.* 3:469–472.

Lenhoff, H.M. (1969). pH profile of a peptide receptor. *Comp. Biochem. Physiol.* 28:571–586.

Lenhoff, H.M. (1968). Behavior, hormones, and Hydra. *Sci.* 161:434–442.

Lentz, T.L. (1968). *Primitive Nervous Systems.* Yale University Press, New Haven.

Liu, Y., and Braud, W.G. (1974). Modification of learning and memory in goldfish through the use of stimulant and depressant drugs. *Psychopharmacologia.* 35:99–112.

Lovell, K.L., and Eisenstein, E.M. (1973). Dark avoidance learning and memory disruption by carbon dioxide in cockroaches. *Physiol. Behavior.* 10:835–840.

Ludány, G., Vajda, J., Ricó, J., and Tu Vu, H. (1958). 5-hydroxytryptamin und die Phagozytose der Leukozyten. *Acta Physiol. Acad. Scientiar. Hungar.* 14:371–373.

Marrone, R.L., Pray, S.L., and Bridges C.C. (1966). Norepinephrine elicitation of aggressive display responses in *Betta splendens. Psychonom. Sci.* 5:207–208.

Mercier, J., and Dessaigne, S. (1971). Influence exercée par la gallamine sur la motricité et les réflexes de la Mante religieuse et du Scorpion. *Compt. Rend. Sociét. Biol.* 165:1368–1371.

Mercier, J., and Dessaigne, S. (1970). Influence exercée par quelques drogues psycholeptiques sur le comportement du Scorpion (*Androctonus australis* Hector) *Compt. Rend. Sociét. Biol.* 164:341–345.

Mirolli, M., and Welsh, J.H. (1964). The effects of reserpine and LSD on molluscs, in *Comparative Neurochemistry.* D. Richter, ed. Pergamon Press, Oxford. pp. 433–443.

Misslin, R., Ropartz, P., and Mandel, P. (1976). Action of Di-n-propylacetate on the spontaneous and acquired behaviour in goldfish, mice, and rats. *Pharmacol. Biochem. Behav.* 4:643–646.

Murdock, L.L. (1971). Catecholamines in Anthropods—a review. *Comp. Gen. Pharmacol.* 2:254–274.

Neale, J.H., Klinger, P.D., and Agranoff, B.W. (1973a). Camptothecin blocks memory of conditioned avoidance in the goldfish. *Sci.* 179:1243–1245.

Neale, J.H., Klinger, P.D., and Agranoff, B.W. (1973b). Temperature-dependent consolidation of puromycin-susceptible memory in the goldfish. *Behav. Biol.* 9:267–278.

Nelson, L. (1972). Neurochemical control of *Arbacia* sperm motility. *Exper. Cell. Res.* 74:269–274.

Newby, N.A. (1973). Habituation to light and spontaneous activity in the isolated siphon of *Aplysia:* Pharmacological observations. *Comp. Gen. Pharmacol.* 4:91–100.

Nistri, A., and Pepeu, G. (1974). Brain acetylcholine levels and nociceptive threshold in frogs after the administration of morphine, nalorphine, and naloxone. *J. Physiol.* 241:51P–52P.

Oelkers, H.A. (1960). Die Eignung von *Betta splendens* zur Differenzienung psychotroper Mittel. *Arzneimittel-Forsch.* 10:392–395.

Ogilvie, D.M., and Fryer, J.N. (1971). Effect of sodium pentobarbital on the temperature selection response of guppies (*Poecilia reticulata*). *Canad. J. Zool.* 49:949–951.

Ohi, S. (1975): The effects of actinomycin D on the brain RNA synthesis and on the passive avoidance latency in the goldfish. *Japanese Journal of Psychology* 46:191–198.

Ohi, S. (1977): Effects of actinomycin D on brain RNA synthesis and discrimination learning in the goldfish (*Carassius auratus*). *Physiology and Behavior* 19:261–264.

Ohr, E.A. (1976a) Tricaine methanesulfonate-I. pH and its effects on anesthetic potency. *Comp. Biochem. Physiol.* 54C:13–17.

Ohr, E.A. (1976b). Tricaine methanesulfonate-II. Effects on transport of NaCl and $H_2O$. *Comp. Biochem. Physiol.* 54C:19–22.

Olson, R.D., Elder, S.T., and May, J.G. (1973). Effect of magnesium pemoline on the habituation of an innate fear response in *Carassius auratus*. *Behav. Biol.* 9:649–653.

Oshima, K., Gorbman, A., and Shimada, H. (1969). Memory-blocking agents: Effects on olfactory discrimination in homing salmon. *Sci.* 165:86–88.

Oxenkrug, G.F., and Lapin, I.P. (1971). Effect of dimethyl and monomethyl tricyclic antidepressants on central 5-hydroxytryptamine processes in the frog. *J. Pharm. Pharmacol.* 23:971–972.

Peeke, H.V.S., Ellman, G., and Herz, M.J. (1973). Dose dependent alcohol effects on the aggressive behavior of the convict cichlid (*Chichlasoma nigrofasciatum*). *Behav. Biol.* 8:115–122.

Peeke, H.V.S., Peeke, S.C., Avis, H.H., and Ellman, G. (1975). Alcohol, habituation, and the patterning of aggressive responses in a cichlid fish. *Pharmacol. Biochem. Behav.* 3:1031–1036.

Peretz, B., Roth, G.E., and Hulette, J. (1971). Acetylcholine involvement in habituated withdrawal responses in *Aplysia* gill. *Fed. Proc.* 30:375Abs.

Peters, H.M., and Witt, P.N. (1949). Die Wirkung von Substanzen auf den Netzbau der Spinnen. *Experientia.* 5:161–162.

Peters, H.M., Witt, P.N., and Wolff, D. (1950). Die Beeinflussung des Netzbaues der Spinnen durch neurotrope Substanzen. *Zeit. vergleich. Physiol.* 32:29–44.

Petty, F., Bryant, R.C., and Byrne, W.L. (1973). Dose-related facilitation by alcohol of avoidance acquisition in the goldfish. *Pharmacol. Biochem. Behav.* 1:173–176.

Pitman, R.M. (1971). Transmitter substances in insects: A review. *Comp. Gen. Pharmacol.* 2:347–372.

Potts, A., and Bitterman, M.F. (1967). Puromycin and retention in the goldfish. *Sci.* 158:1594–1596.

Raynes, A.E., and Ryback, R.S. (1970). Effects of alcohol and congeners on aggressive response in *Detta splendens*. *Quart. J. Stud. Alc.* Supp. 5:130–135.

Raynes, A.E., Ryback, R., and Ingle, D. (1968). The effect of alcohol of aggression in *Betta splendens*. *Comm. Behav. Biol.* A2:141–146.

Reed, C.F., and Witt, P.N. (1968). Progressive disturbance of spider web geometry caused by two sedative drugs. *Physiol. Behav.* 3:119–124.

Rensch, B., and Dücker, G. (1966). Verzögerung des Vergessens erlernter visueller Aufgaben bei Tieren durch chlorpromazine. *Pflügers Arch. gesamte Physiol.* 289:200–214.

Reynolds, W.W., and Covert, J.B. (1977). Behavioral fever in aquatic ectothermic vertebrates, in *Drugs, Biogenic Amines, and Body Temperature.* K.E. Cooper, P. Lomax, and E. Schönbaum, eds. Karger, Basel. pp. 108–110.

Riege, W.H., and Cherkin, A. (1976). Memory performance after flurothyl treatment in rainbow trout. *Psychopharmacologia* 46:31–35.

Riege, W.H., and Cherkin, A. (1973). Retroactive facilitation of memory in goldfish by flurothyl. *Psychopharmacologia* 30:195–204.

Rosič, N., Lomax, P., and Kovačevič, N. (1974). The toxic and behavioural effects of cholinesterase inhibitor in fish (*Serranus scriba*). *Comp. Gen. Pharmacol.* 5:187–189.

Rozin, P. (1968). The use of poikilothermy in the analysis of behavior, in *The Central Nervous System and Fish Behavior*. D. Ingle, ed. Univ. of Chicago Press, Chicago. pp. 181-192.

Ryback, R.S. (1976). A method to study short-term memory (STM) in the goldfish. *Pharmacol. Biochem. Behav.* 4:489-491.

Ryback, R.S. (1970). The use of fish, especially goldfish, in alcohol research. *Quart. J. Stud. Alc.* 31:162-166.

Ryback, R.S. (1969a). State-dependent or "dissociated" learning with alcohol in the goldfish. *Quart. J. Stud. Alc.* 30:598-608.

Ryback, R.S. (1969b). The use of goldfish as a model for alcohol amnesia in man. *Quart. J. Stud. Alc.* 30:877-882.

Ryback, R.S. (1969c). Effect of ethanol, bourbon, and various ethanol levels on Y-maze learning in the goldfish. *Psychopharmacologia.* 14:305-314.

Ryback, R.S., and Ingle, D. (1970). Effect of ethanol and bourbon on Y-maze learning and shock avoidance in the goldfish. *Quart. J. Stud. Alc.* Supp. 5:136-141.

Ryback, R. S., Percarpio, B., and Vitale, J. (1969). Equilibration and metabolism of ethanol in the goldfish. *Nat.* 222:1068-1070.

Sacchi, U., and Gianniotti, G. (1956a). Inibizione dell'iniziative motrice del pesce (*Carassius auratus*) da 5-HT. *Boll. Soc. Ital. Biol. Sper.* 32:175-177.

Sacchi, U., and Gianniotti, G. (1956b). Antagonismo tra LSD e 5-HT sulla iniziativa motrice del pesce (*Carassius auratus*). *Boll. Soc. Ital. Biol. sper.* 32:177-179.

Sahagian, D.E., and Ingle, D.J. (1977). The effects of amphetamine on maze learning by goldfish. *Psychopharmacol.* 53:319-320.

Sakharov, D.A. (1970). Cellular aspects of invertebrate neuropharmacology. *Ann. Rev. Pharmacol.* 10:335-352.

Schoel, W.M., and Agranoff, B.W. (1972). The effect of puromycin on retention of conditioned cardiac deceleration in the goldfish. *Behav. Biol.* 7:553-565.

Shashoua, V.E. (1968a). RNA changes in goldfish brain during learning. *Nat.* 217:238-240.

Shashoua, V.E. (1968b). The relation of RNA metabolism in the brain to learning in the goldfish, in *Central Nervous System and Fish Behavior*. D. Ingle, ed. Univ. of Chicago Press, Chicago. pp. 203-213.

Smit, G.L. and Hattingh, J. (1979): Anaesthetic potency of MS 222 and neutralized MS 222 as studied in three freshwater fish species. *Comparative Biochemistry and Physiology* 62C:237-241.

Springer, A.D., and Agranoff, B.W. (1976). Electroconvulsive chock- or puromycin-induced retention deficits in goldfish given two active-avoidance sessions. *Behav. Biol.* 18:309-324.

Stahl, S.M., Narotzky, R., Boshes, B., and Zeller, E.A. (1971). Einfluss des zerebralen Amin-Stoffwechsels auf das Gedächtnis des Goldfisches. *Naturwissenschaften.* 58:628-629.

Stefano, G.B., and Catapane, E.J. (1977). The effect of temperature acclimation on monoamine metabolism. *J. Pharmacol. Exper. Therapeut.* 203:449-456.

Stenger, V.G., and Maren, T.H. (1974). The pharmacology of MS222 (ethyl-m-aminobenzoate) in *Squalus acanthias*. *Comp. Gen. Pharmacol.* 5:23-35.

Tamano, M. (1960). Effect of some drugs acting on the central and autonomic nervous system and of some mitotic inhibitors on the growth and metamorphosis of the silkworm, and on the properties of its cocoon and thread. *Fol. pharmacolog. Jap.* 56:38.

Tarchalska, B., Kostowski, W., Markowska, L., and Markiewicz, L. (1975). On the role of serotonin in aggressive behaviour of ants genus *Formica*. *Pol. J. Pharmacol. Pharm.* 27:237-239.

Toğrol, B.B., Ormanli, M., and Cantez, E. (1966). The effects of chemicals on the general behavior, regeneration, and the learning capacity of planaria. *Polycelis tenuis* (Ijima) and *Dugesia lugubris* (Schmidt). *Rev. Fac. Sci. Istambul.* 31:167-181.

Ungar, G., Desiderio, D.M., and Parr, W. (1972). Isolation, identification, and synthesis of a specific-behavior-inducing brain peptide. *Nat.* 238:198-202.

Valzelli, L. (1974). 5-hydroxytryptamine in aggressiveness. *Adv. Biochem. Psychopharmacol.* 11:255–263.

Vowles, D.M. (1964). Olfactory learning and brain lesions in the wood ant (*Formica rufa*). *J. Comp. Physiol. Psychol.* 58:105–111.

Walaszek, E.J., and Abood, L.G. (1956). Effect of tranquilizing drugs on fighting response of Siamese fighting fish. *Sci.* 124:440–441.

Waldes, V. (1938). Uber die chemische Beeinflussung des Rhythmus und der Retraktionsdauer der Cirren von *Balanus perforatus. Zeit. vergleich. Physiol.* 26:347–361.

Weischer, M.-L. (1966): Einfluss von Anorektica der Amphetamin-Reihe auf das Verhalten des Siamesischen Kampffisches *Betta splendens. Arzneimittel-Forschung* 16:1310–1311.

Weischer, M.-L. (1969): Über die antiaggressive Wirkung von Lithium. *Psychopharmacologia* 15:245–254.

Welch, A.S., and Welch, B.L. (1968). Effect of stress and para-chlorophenylalanine upon brain serotonin, 5-hydroxyindoleacetic acid and catecholamines in grouped and isolated mice. *Biochem. Pharmacol.* 17:699–708.

Wilson, W.L., Darcy, J.M., and Haralson, J.V. (1970). Reserpine and conditioned suppression in the fish *Tilaphia h. macrocephala. Psychonom. Sci.* 20:47–49.

Witt, P.N. (1971). Drugs alter web-building of spiders: A review and evaluation. *Behav. Sci.* 16:98–113.

Witt, P.N. (1956). *Die Wirkung von Substanzen auf den Netzbau der Spinne als biologischer Test.* Springer, Heidelberg.

Witt, P.N. (1955). Die Wirkung einer einmaligen Gabe von Largactil auf den Netzbau der Spinne *Zilla-x-notata. Monat. Psychiat. Neurol.* 129:123–128.

Witt, P.N. (1951). d-Lysergsäure-diethylamid (LSD 25) im Spinnentest. *Experientia.* 7:310–311.

Witt, P.N., Breitschneider L., and Boris, A.P. (1961). Sensitivity to D-amphetamine in spiders after iproniazid and imipramine. *J. Pharmacol. Exper. Therapeut.* 132:183–192.

Witt, P.N., Reed, C.F., and Peakall, D.B. (1968). *A Spider's Web. Problems in Regulatory Biology.* Springer, New York.

Wolff, D., and Hempel, U. (1951). Versuche über die Beeinflussung des Netzbaues von *Zilla-x-notata* durch Pervitin, Scopolamin und Strychnin. *Zeit. vergleich. Physiol.* 33:497–528.

Current Developments in Psychopharmacology, Volume 6
© 1981, Spectrum Publications, Inc.

CHAPTER 2

# BEHAVIORAL EFFECTS OF OPIATES: A PHARMACOGENETIC ANALYSIS

ALBERTO OLIVERIO
CLAUDIO CASTELLANO

## A. INDIVIDUAL AND SPECIES DIFFERENCES IN DRUG REACTIVITY

A number of experiments carried out in recent years, have emphasized individual differences in reactivity to many psychotropic agents, both in humans and in laboratory animals. This may be due to differences in the rate of absorption, distribution, metabolism, or excretion of drugs; or to differences in the sensitivity of target systems to compounds acting at the central nervous system (CNS) level.

In particular, as far as drug metabolism is concerned, it must be observed that different animal species vary both in the kind of enzyme systems they possess and in their quantitative distribution (Koppanyi and Avery, 1966). Williams (1962) has illustrated the clear differences existing in the enzyme patterns of different species: Men, for example, are able to form conjugated glucuronides, to acetylate aromatic amines, etc., while cats are defective in glucuronyl transferase and dogs do not acetylate arylamines.

A number of genetically determined differences in drug sensitivity due to abnormal enzymatic pathways have been recognized to account for slow or fast inactivation of a great number of drugs, such as isoniazid, anticoagulants, barbiturates, or antidepressant agents (Kalow, 1966; Koppanyi and Avery, 1966). It has been demonstrated, for example, that barbital is retained for a longer time in the brains of cats and dogs than that of rabbits, a fact which might account for differences in response to barbiturate administration among these animal species. Similarly, Quinn et al. (1954)

have shown that the activity of the liver enzyme that oxidizes hexobarbital to ketobarbital is high in species in which the drug has a short duration of action, and low in those in which the drug acts for a longer time. After injecting a dose of 100 mg/kg of hexobarbital into mice, rabbits, and rats, and a dose of 50 mg/kl into dogs, the order of sleeping time recorded in their experiments was: mice: 12 min; rabbits: 49 min; rats: 95 min; dogs: 260 min. The half-life was shown to parallel the sleeping time and to be correlated with enzyme activity.

A number of findings suggest that the amount of substrate present in a given species may account for the effects of drugs that inhibit enzyme activity, such as cholinesterase (ChE) or monoamino-oxidase (MAO) inhibitors. Species differences in the effects of MAO inhibitors may be ascribed, for example, to large species variations in the rate of catecholamine synthesis. In fact, it has been shown that iproniazid and pargyline do not increase the levels of brain catecholamines in dogs and cats (although 5-hydroxytryptophane levels are elevated), while the same drugs enhance the levels of NA and 5H tryptamine in the brains of rabbits or cats (Gillette, 1965). It seems clear that interspecies or intraspecies differences in drug responses may be ascribed both to differences in plasma levels (quantitative variations in the amounts of a particular chemical), and to variations in the ratio between two mediators. Meier (1963) reports, for example, that the ratio of NA to A, which is quite constant in most animal species, may vary between individual cats from 13 to 91 percent.

## B.  SPECIES DIFFERENCES IN THE REACTIVITY TO OPIATES

As far as opiates are concerned, interspecies differences in sensitivity to their effects have been reported by a number of investigators. Among mammals, for example, morphine exerts a narcotic effect in dogs, rabbits, guinea pigs, and rats; psychic excitement follows morphine treatment in cats and horses, while morphine-injected rams, goats, and pigs show an increased motor activity (Criswell and Levit, 1975). In humans, behavioral excitement occurs following morphine administration, but it is generally masked by a stronger depressive effect (Criswell and Levitt, 1975). As far as the toxicity of the opiates is concerned, differences have also been reported among different animal species, these toxic effects being higher, for example, in carnivores than in rodents.

### 1.   Opiates and Behavior: Biochemical Correlates

In recent years a number of investigations have been concerned with the effects of morphine on the behavior of animals. The effects of opiates on analgesia and running activity, the development of tolerance to narcotic drug administrations, etc., have been extensively studied and a number of biochemical correlations have been suggested. In this respect, a number of studies suggest that cholinergic mechanisms at the CNS level may explain some mechanisms related to tolerance and abstinence in rats and mice (Domino and Wilson, 1973; Jhamandas and Dickinson, 1973). However, serotoninergic mechanisms also seem to play a role in morphine-induced analgesia and in opiate tolerance, or physical dependence (Cheney and Goldstein, 1971; Samanin and Valzelli, 1972; Way et al., 1973; Yarbrough et al., 1973).

By using different measures of locomotor activity, it has been shown that morphine exerts a stimulating effect in mice (Shuster et al., 1963; Goldstein and Sheehan, 1969). The effects of morphine on locomotor activity, together with the analgesic effects of the opiates have been related by some authors (Giarman and Pepeu, 1962; Jhamandas et al., 1970; Sharkawi, 1970; Pepeu et al., 1971) to a reduction of the release of acetylcholine at the central cholinergic synapses level, or to alterations in brain catecholamines content and turnover (Rethy et al., 1971; Buxbaum et al., 1973; Villarreal et al., 1973).

A number of behavioral investigations have been concerned with the onset of tolerance to the effects of opiates following both acute and chronic treatments.

## 2.  Opiates: Acute Effects

The development of acute tolerance to morphine-induced locomotor activity and analgesia has been, in particular, extensively studied in mice and rats.

Experiments dealing with the development (and loss) of tolerance to the analgesic effect of single injections of morphine in rats have shown that acute tolerance is a long-lasting phenomenon, and its development is blocked by protein synthesis and nucleic acid inhibitors (Cochin and Kornetsky, 1964; Lotti et al., 1966). In this respect, findings obtained by Cox et al. (1968), have moreover demonstrated that some degree of tolerance develops within 3 to 4 hours after the start of an infusion of morphine, diamorphine, and etorphine, and that the simultaneous infusion of actinomycin D (which inhibits protein synthesis) prevents the development of tolerance.

The development of tolerance after the administration of morphine at 4 hour intervals for 2 days was studied by Huidobro and Huidobro (1973) in newborn and young Sprague Dawley rats. Tolerance was measured by means of the hot-plate method. The authors have demonstrated that a positive correlation exists between loss of sensitivity to morphine and age. Their experiments have also emphasized that the development of acute tolerance to morphine-induced analgesia does not depend on the stage of development of the rat, since tolerance developed at all the ages tested (16-, 25-, and 38-day-old animals).

### 3. Opiates: Chronic Effects

As far as chronic morphine treatments are concerned, it has been shown that repeated administrations of the drug may affect a wide range of behavioral measures in animals. Seevers and Deneau (1963) have demonstrated, for example, that chronic administrations of morphine in a variety of species are followed by development of tolerance to the central nervous system depressant effects of the opiate. More recently, Rethy et al. (1971) have shown that tolerance to both the stimulating effect on locomotor activity and to the brain catecholamine-depleting effect develops in mice after repeated administrations of morphine and related analgesics. In these experiments, tolerance was produced by injecting either morphine (100 mg/kg) or levorphanol (56 mg/kg) every 6 hours. The same authors have shown that pretreatment with naloxone prevents the effects of morphine and related analgesics upon both catecholamine contents and locomotor activity.

The development of physical dependence on morphine through pellets implanted subcutaneously has proved to be a fruitful method in the investigations of the effects of opiates on behavior. Recently Bläsig, et al. (1974) have utilized this technique in rats by inducing different degrees of dependence in the animals, (1) by varying the dosage, (2) frequency of implantation, and (3) duration of exposure to morphine. Withdrawal was precipitated by injections of morphine antagonists (e.g., levallorphan). When withdrawal was precipitated, Bläsig and co-workers observed the appearance of various signs, some of which became progressively more pronounced when dependence got stronger, or the dose of antagonist was increased. On the contrary, other signs showed a maximal frequency at the lower degrees of dependence, or after the administration of the lower doses of antagonist, and decreased or disappeared when the degree of dependence became higher, or the dose of antagonist was further increased. The authors have thus classified these signs into "recessive" signs, such as writing and wet dog shaking, which decline when "dominant" signs, such as jumping, flying, and teeth-chattering increase.

Further experiments based on the same technique (pellets implanted subcutaneously) have shown that the administration of low doses of d-amphetamine, cocaine, and L-DOPA shortly before precipitating withdrawal by levallorphan induced a dose-dependent increase of "dominant" signs (i.e., jumping), and a decrease of "recessive" signs (i.e., wet dog shaking) (Herz et al., 1974). In the same research, activation of adrenergic or dopaminergic mechanisms based on the use of desipramine or apomorphine induced an increase in the intensity of withdrawal, while catecholamines depletion (with $\mu$ MT) led to a loss in the effectiveness of the apomorphine treatment. Therefore, it was concluded that both dopamine and noradrenaline (and especially NA) are involved in the manifestation of the morphine withdrawal syndrome.

Recently, Laschka et al. (1976) have also identified the sites of action of morphine involved in the development of physical dependence in rats. In these experiments, morphine withdrawal was precipitated by the injection of various morphine antagonists into restricted parts of the ventricular system or by microinjections of levallorphan into specific brain areas of rats made dependent on morphine by repeated pellet implantations. The results led to the conclusion that brain structures located in the anterior part of the floor of the fourth ventricle and/or caudal parts of the periaqueductal gray matter are important sites of action for the development of physical dependence on morphine.

## C. THE USE OF INBRED STRAINS IN PHARMACOGENETIC INVESTIGATIONS

In recent years, the large number of genetic experiments on the laboratory mouse has resulted in many lines and inbred strains (Staats, 1972), and has provided much information on the neurophysiological and behavioral maturation of this species. Large individual differences have been observed for the weights and sizes of some cerebral structures (Wimer et al., 1971), the levels of cholinergic and adrenergic mediators (Ebel et al., 1973; Mandel et al., 1973), and the electroencephalographic patterns (Valatx et al., 1972). The existence of these differences makes the laboratory mouse a very useful tool for pharmacogenetic analyses. One reason to use inbred strains is related to the extreme behavioral homogeneity of the individuals belonging to the same line; the second reason is related to the difference among behavioral traits characterizing each strain.

When a number of behavioral measures are considered, large differences are in fact evident among inbred strains of mice (McClearn et al., 1970; Lindzey et al., 1971; Wahlsten, 1972). Similarly, drugs acting upon different behavioral responses are apt to be strain-dependent in their effects: These effects were correlated to qualitative or quantitative strain differences in specific enzyme content, to altered mechanisms of excretion or liver metabolism, or to different patterns of action at the brain level.

### 1. CNS Depressant and Tranquillizing Agents

Differences in the rate of inactivation in the liver might account for the large differences in sleeping time evident between BALB/c and CBA mice, injected with the same dose of nembutal (Brown, 1959). Strain differences in a variety of behaviors related to alcohol consumption have also been reported (Eriksson, 1969; Fuller, 1964; McClearn and Rodgers, 1959) (C57BL/6 mice showed high preference for a 10 percent ethanol solution; DBA/2 strain avoided the solution almost completely). Comparisons of high and low preferring strains by a number of investigators have provided the evidence that the activities of the liver enzymes, alcohol dehydrogenase and aldehyde dehydrogenase, are related to spontaneous preference. The role of the levels of "kinetic drive" in the dose response curves of a given drug has been underlined by Fuller (1966, 1970). This author tested four inbred strains of mice and found that strain differences in avoidance learning were related to variations in strength of kinetic drive. He observed that, while no association was found between the effectiveness of chlorpromazine (CPZ) and genotype, the dose-response curves with chlordiazepoxide (CDP) did vary with respect to the mean levels of activity of the strains considered. For CDP, the values of the regression coefficient for the strains ranged from +26.5 in the C57BL/6J mice to –133.7 in the DBA/2J mice. In general, CDP appeared to enhance responding in the least active strains and decrease it in the more active strains.

Strain-dependent effects of CDP on avoidance behavior of mice have also been evident in some findings of Sansone and Messeri (1973). In their experiments, the dose that induced a 50 percent impairment of performance in a previously acquired avoidance task has been about two times higher in the SEC/1ReJ strain than in the BALB/c mice.

## 2.  Cholinergic and Adrenergic Agents

In a more sophisticated behavioral pattern, such as avoidance learning, clear differences in strain reactivity with regard to the effects of psychoactive agents have been found in a number of researches. Bovet, Bovet-Nitti and Oliverio (1969) have demonstrated, for example, that the magnitude of the performance impairments following arecoline administration in this experimental situation is strain-dependent.

Among the many other investigations emphasizing the role of the genetic makeup in modulating the effects of drugs on behavior are the studies of Bovet et al. (1966) with nicotine, showing facilitation of avoidance learning in low learners and impairment in high-learner strains following the administration of this drug. Further experiments have supported the hypothesis that nicotine facilitates acquisition and retention processes (Oliverio, 1968; Evangelista et al., 1970).

Studies recently carried out in our laboratory (Oliverio and Castellano, 1973) have considered the sensitivity to metrazol-induced seizures, and the effects of adrenergic and cholinergic agents on behavior in DBA/2J,

C57BL/6J, and SEC1/ReJ mice. A first set of experiments showed, in agreement with previous findings (Schlesinger and Griek, 1970) that DBA and SEC strains display lower metrazol thresholds than C57 animals. In this case, when the hybrids C57×SEC were considered, they resembled the SEC phenotype, while the C57×DBA mice resembled the C57 strain.

In a second set of experiments, the effects of an adrenergic (amphetamine) and a cholinergic agent (scopolamine) on the exploratory activity of the different strains were assessed as compared with saline-injected mice. The results showed, in agreement with previous findings (van Abeelen, 1966), that exploratory activity differed in control mice among strains. The number of crossings was, in fact, two times higher in C57 strain than in the other two lines. In offspring of the C57 mice, it showed a low or high exploratory activity, depending on whether it derived from a cross with SEC or with DBA.

When the responses to amphetamine and to scopolamine were investigated, differences also appeared among the strains tested: both drugs reduced the activity in the C57 mice, while the number of crossings was increased in the other two strains. The responses of the C57×SEC hybrids to amphetamine and scopolamine were similar to those of the SEC mice. When the crossings C57×DBA were examined, however, the usual pattern of dominance was absent. Amphetamine, in fact, decreased the number of crossings (like it did in the C57 strain), while scopolamine enhanced the activity of the C57×DBA mice, as was observed in the DBA strain.

These findings indicate that, as far as the response to amphetamine is concerned, the C57 genotype is dominant over the DBA, while it is recessive with respect to the DBA genotype when the effects of scopolamine are considered.

## D. A PHARMACOGENETIC APPROACH TO OPIATES

In recent years, the genetic approach has also proved to be very fruitful in the study of the effects of opiates on behavior in mice.

Eriksson and Kiianmaa (1971) have analyzed the susceptibility to morphine addiction in two inbred strains of mice (CBA/Ca and C57BL). In their experiments, mice were given daily morphine injections for 3 weeks. This was followed by a 5-day forcing stage, when the animals were given only aqueous morphine solutions to drink, and a 2-day abstinence period. The mice were then given a free choice between tap water and aqueous morphine solution for 1 week. Morphine consumption was used as the measure of phenotype. The results showed that morphine consumption is higher in the C57BL mice than in the CBA.

In another investigation, by using CF₁ and CFW strains of mice,

Gebhart and Mitchell (1973) showed the existence of strain differences in the analgesic response to morphine (measured with the hot plate). In their experiments, morphine was found to be 16 times more efficacious in the $CF_1$ mice than in the CFW strain.

A number of recent studies have demonstrated that C57BL/6J and DBA/2J mice are a very useful tool to study the effects of opiates on behavior. The genetic approach with these strains seems to be a useful method in order to assess which biochemical systems are involved in the various behavioral effects following morphine administration. Differences in behavior and brain chemicals have been demonstrated between these strains in basal conditions.

With regard to behavior, it has been shown that C57 strain is character-ized by high levels of exploratory activity and lower levels of avoidance and maze learning than DBA mice (Bovet et al., 1969; Elias, 1970; Sprott, 1971; Oliverio et al., 1973; Renzi and Sansone, 1971).

Biochemical investigations have shown that the DBA strain, as com-pared with the C57 strain, is characterized by higher acetylcholinesterase (AChe) and lower cholineacetyltransferase (ChA) activities in the temporal lobe (Ebel et al., 1973; Mandel et al., 1973); and, for the adrenergic system, by higher levels of NA in the pons and the medulla oblongata (Kempf et al., 1974; Mack et al., 1973). Clear differences between the regional brain NA turnover have also been demonstrated between those two strains by Eleftheriou (1971).

## 1. Effects of Opiates on Analgesia and Motor Activity of Inbred Strains

On the grounds of the behavioral and biochemical differences reported above, some studies have been carried out with the C57 and DBA strains in our laboratory, dealing with the effects of opiates on behavior.

In the first group of experiments, we have determined the sensitivity of C57BL/6J, DBA/2J, and BALB/cJ mice to morphine-induced motor activity and analgesia (Oliverio and Castellano, 1974b). The locomotor activity was measured with toggle floor boxes, and the effects on analgesia with the hot-plate method (Eddy and Leimback, 1953), as modified by Goldstein and Sheehan (1969). The results showed that, regarding locomo-tor activity, the strains tested were clearly different when the morphine-induced "running fit" was considered. A threefold average increase was, in fact, evident in the C57 strain following morphine (or heroin) administra-tion, while no effect appeared when the opiates were injected into the DBA mice. The BALB strain, characterized by high levels of avoidance and low levels of locomotor activity in basal conditions, showed a twofold increment of activity following opiates administration. (See Figure 1.)

As far as the effects of the opiates on analgesia were concerned, the

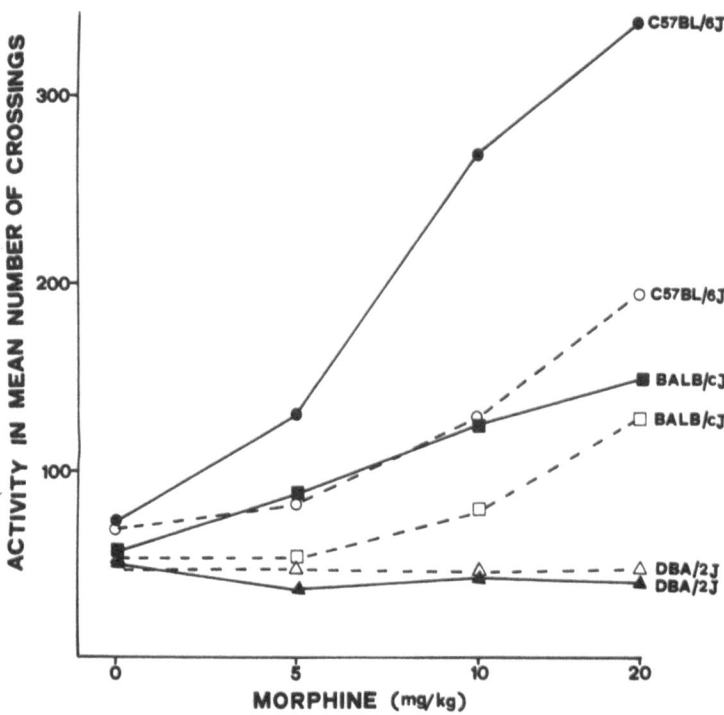

**Figure 1.**    Effects of different doses of morphine on the running activity of normal (solid lines) and tolerant (broken lines) mice. Each group consisted of 10 mice tested 30 min after injection of morphine (Oliverio and Castellano, 1974b).

pattern of reactivity was completely opposite to that observed in the activity measures. In fact, the analgesic effect was less evident in the C57 mice, which had been very sensitive to the stimulating properties of the drugs on activity; while in DBA (and BALB) mice, the analgesia was very high (See Figure 2.) Therefore it was evident that the effects of opiates on both analgesia and running activity were strain-dependent. It was also evident that they were likely to imply two different sites of action, in that they were clearly dissociated, a negative correlation between the degree of running and analgesic responses caused by the opiates being clearly evident in the strains considered.

## 2.    Genetic Analysis of Morphine-Induced Analgesia and Running Fit

When the genetic analysis of the effects of morphine on running and analgesia was extended to the $F_1$ hybrids of the three strains tested (Castellano and Oliverio, 1975), the experiments showed that the performance of the C57×DBA and the C57×BALB mice were similar to those of

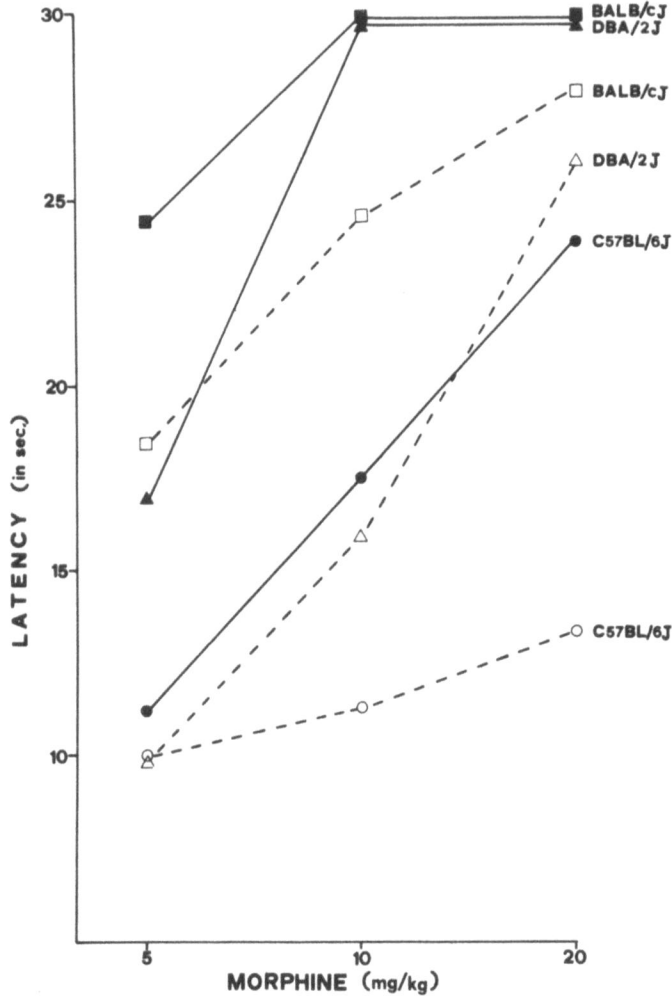

**Figure 2.** Morphine-induced analgesia in normal (solid lines) and tolerant (broken lines) mice. The animals were tested 30 min after the injection with different doses of opiate (Oliverio and Castellano, 1974b).

the C57 strain, thus showing a dominance of the C57 strain over the other two. In addition, the inheritance of morphine analgesia seemed to be regulated by incomplete dominance, in that the performances of C57×BALB and C57×DBA mice were very similar to that of the C57 strain.

## 3. Behavioral Effects of Opiates: A Neurophysiological Approach

According to a number of investigations, different models might account for the effects of opiates on running activity and analgesia. As previously mentioned in this chapter, catecholamine depletion seems to be associated with running-fit syndrome in mice (and decrease in serotonin levels seems to facilitate it) (Cheney and Goldstein, 1971; Hollinger, 1969; Rethy et al., 1971); cholinergic factors seem, instead, to play an important role in opiate-induced analgesia and abstinence (Cheney and Goldstein, 1971; Domino and Wilson, 1973; Jhamandas and Dickinson, 1973). It may be thus suggested that the biochemical differences existing between C57 and DBA mice might be responsible for the strain-dependent effects of opiates and for the dissociation between the effects of morphine on running and analgesic behavior evident in our experiments.

The role played by the neurophysiological systems and by brain chemicals in the effects of opiates on these two measures in C57 and DBA mice has been clarified by further experiments, through the analysis of the interaction between septal lesions and morphine-induced running fit and analgesia in these two strains (Castellano et al., 1975). Some investigations have shown the relationship existing between opiate receptors in the brain and neurotransmitters, and that opiate receptor sites are already associated with the limbic system (a critical area for eliciting analgesia) (Kuhar et al., 1973; Herz et al., 1970; Wey et al., 1973.) The experiments by Castellano et al. (1975) have demonstrated that septal lesions have no effect on the morphine-induced running fit, while analgesia may be antagonized by these lesions in both strains. By pretreating mice with $\alpha$-methyl-p-tyrosine ($\alpha$MT), inhibition of the synthesis of NA resulted in these experiments in a marked reduction of the locomotor activity of all mice tested.

Since it is evident from the literature that lesions of the septal area result in a decreased cholinergic input to other regions of the limbic system (Kuhar et al., 1973; Srebro et al., 1973), these data suggest that, as far as morphine-induced analgesia is concerned, a reduction of the cholinergic activity in the limbic system, due to septal lesions, interferes with the effects of morphine on analgesic behavior. The fact that septal lesions decreased morphine-induced analgesia but not the running fit, while $\alpha$MT antagonized the effects of the opiate on locomotor activity but not the effects on analgesia, may lead to the conclusion that the same biochemical and neurophysiological model cannot explain the effects of the opiate on the two measures considered. It may also be argued that the limbic system modulates morphine-induced analgesia in the mouse, but not the effects of morphine on locomotor activity.

Experiments carried out by Oliverio (1975) have shown that C57 and DBA mice are also different when their electrocorticographic (ECoG) response to morphine administration is considered. In these experiments, the only difference between the ECoG's of the saline-injected animals of the two strains was evident in the sleep recordings; during sleep, in fact, larger spindles appeared in the DBA than in the C57 mice. Regarding the effect of the opiate, the ECoG of the DBA mice was not affected by morphine administration, while a single acute injection of morphine was followed (3 to 10 minutes after injection) by an increase in voltage and the appearance of slow waves and spindles in the C57 strain. This change lasted for as long as 45 to 60 minutes and was accompanied by behavioral activation.

In a second set of experiments, the effect of septal lesions on ECoG patterns and running activity as investigated. (See Figure 3.) It was evident that neither the ECoG nor the running response was modified by septal lesions; the lesions reduced only the analgesic response to the opiate administration in the DBA mice. These results suggest: (1) the existence of a correlation between behavioral activation and sleep-like ECoG patterns, and (2) the existence of a similarity between the effects of the anticholinergic drugs and those of morphine, since a dissociation between ECoG and behavior became evident following morphine administration. The results also confirm the hypothesis that locomotor or other excitatory patterns,

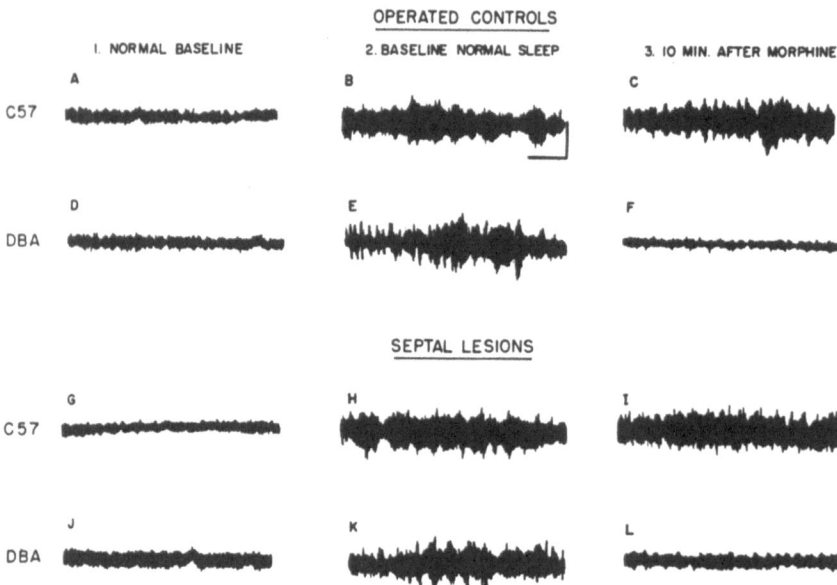

**Figure 3.** Effects of a single injection of morphine on the EEG tracing recorded from the cortex in normal mice (operated controls) and in mice with lesions of the septum. Samples of polygraphic recording during waking (1. normal baseline), slow wave sleep (2. baseline normal sleep), and after the injection of morphine (20 mg/kg) in C57BL/6J and DBA/2J mice (3). The normal sleep EEG (B) and that after morphine injection (C) are similar in the C57BL/6J strain. However, in DBA mice, the waking EEG (D) and that after morphine injection (F) are similar. Septal lesions do not produce any major modification of the effects of morphine on the EEG patterns (Oliverio, 1975).

rather than the analgesic effects of morphine, are possibly correlated to the electroencephalographic (EEG) responses to the opiate administration.

## 4. Behavioral Effects of Pharmacological Combinations with Opiates

Further studies have emphasized the role played by the genetic makeup in modulating the effects of different combinations of opiates with other drugs on the locomotor activity of mice (Castellano et al., 1976). The combinations of heroin with ethanol, amphetamine, or strychnine, have, in fact, affected the motor responses in C57 and DBA mice, and the type of responses were different, depending on the strain. In particular, the combinations of heroin plus amphetamine and heroin plus ethanol were followed by a clear stimulation of the locomotor activity of the DBA mice; while the activity of the C57 mice was stimulated only by the strychnine plus heroin mixture. When the toxicity of the heroin plus strychnine combination was analyzed, it was evident that this combination was always characterized by a higher toxicity, in comparison to the toxicity of heroin alone —DL 50 $_{heroin\ alone}$: 200 mg/kg in the C57 strain and 250 mg/kg in the DBA; DL 50 $_{comb.}$: 150 mg/kg (C57) and 100 mg/kg (DBA).

These results seem to be important for their clinical and toxicological implications, since many lethal incidents attributed to an overdose of heroin might be instead ascribed to the use of adulterants, which enhance the effects of the opiate.

## E. DOPAMINERGIC AND CHOLINERGIC MECHANISMS IN RELATION TO STRAIN DIFFERENCES IN OPIATES EFFECT

With regard to the effects of morphine on locomotor activity and analgesia in DBA and C57 mice, recent experiments (Trabucchi et al., 1976) have suggested that they may be related to well-established biochemical differences at the brain level.

According to these authors, two separate neurochemical patterns seem to be related to the effects of morphine on running activity and analgesia. The findings have shown that in the C57 mice, whose activity patterns are considerably stimulated following the opiate administration, striatal adenylate cyclase is more stimulated by dopamine than in the DBA strain. It has also been demonstrated that striatal dopaminergic neurons are activated mainly in C57 mice. According to the authors, 3-Methoxy-Tyramine and c AMP are increased by morphine administration only in the C57 strain. Also, morphine-induced analgesia in the DBA strain seems to implicate cholinergic pathways, since a decrement in the turnover rate of acetylcholine was evident in the limbic structures only in this strain following morphine administration. In the same study, a decrease in the turnover rate of acetylcholine was observed in the striatum of the C57 mice, as a consequence of the activation of the turnover rate of dopamine following morphine administration.

Therefore, Trabucchi et al. (1976) suggest that the striatal dopaminergic system may be involved in the running fit, which follows the opiate administration, since striatal dopaminergic neurons are activated, and the increment in motor activity is antagonized in the C57 strain by antidopaminergic agents. A number of recent experiments also indicate that the levels and turnovers of endorphins are under genetic control (Reggiani et al., 1980); this fact is also supported by recent experiments indicating a differential effect of d-aminoacids (d-Aa) in C57 and DBA mice (Alleva et al., 1980).

## F. OPIATES ADMINISTRATION: ENVIRONMENTAL FACTORS

Recently, it has been suggested that environmental factors play an important role in determining the stimulating effects of morphine, and that the genetic mechanisms are not the sole source of variation when the individual reactivity to opiates is considered (Oliverio and Castellano, 1974). The experiments were carried out with C57BL/6J mice, whose activity was recorded in toggle floor boxes.

The first group of mice was injected with morphine, and a threefold increase in activity was evident, as compared with saline-injected controls. To test the effects of past experience on the effect of the opiate, another group was adapted to the apparatus, injected with morphine immediately after the end of the 25-minute session, and tested again. The activity of this group was not enhanced, in relation to the control group, showing that past experience modifies the effects of the opiate on behavior.

In another set of experiments, the animals were first adapted to the apparatus without drugs. Six hours later, they were subjected to a second 25-minute test; and, at the end of this session, they were injected with saline, or morphine, and were immediately retested during a third 25-minute session. The experience of these animals was thus more consolidated than in the previous schedule, and their activity was completely blocked. However, when the animals were removed and returned to their home cages, very high levels of locomotor activity were evident. After a few minutes, they were tested again in the toggle floor boxes, and a high level of activity was evident under these conditions. It was thus concluded that exploration of a different environment was followed by the running fit in the same experienced animals in which the injection of morphine previously resulted in a complete block of their activity.

The same change in the activity pattern (block→running fit) was induced in experienced animals by either switching off the 40-watt lamp normally lighted in the cabin 1 meter above the apparatus, or by spraying a solution of eugenol inside the cabin at the end of the morphine session. (See Figure 4.)

The importance of sensory inputs and experience in modulating the effects of the opiate were shown by a further series of experiments. In these studies, mice were subjected to functional decortication, and morphine injection was followed by clear excitatory effects.

The results of these investigations stress the importance of the environment in influencing the action of the centrally acting drugs. They may also have a number of implications at the human level, suggesting the importance of a number of "social drugs" in man, depending on his social environment.

## G. SUMMARY

A number of studies are reviewed in relation to a pharmacogenetic approach to the effects of opiates. The behavioral effects of morphine and heroin in different species or strains of animals are considered. In particular, a number of behavioral, neurophysiological, and biochemical correlates of the opiates in different inbred strains of mice are cited.

Recent studies concerning the effects of opiates on behavior have utilized the C57BL/6J and the DBA/2J strains, which are characterized by different brain levels and turnover of cholinergic and adrenergic mediators. It has been shown that the effects of opiates on running activity and on analgesia are strain-dependent, and a negative correlation is evident between the two measures in the strains considered. Experiments carried out on mice with septal lesions and on normal mice have confirmed that the motor and analgesic effects of morphine in the mouse are two distinct phenomena, which may be explained through different neurophysiological and biochemical models. Differences between the strains considered have also been observed when the ECoG response to morphine administration has been investigated. The results of these experiments have suggested:

1. The existence of a correlation between behavioral activation and sleep-like ECoG patterns.

2. The existence of a similarity between the effects of the anticholinergic drugs and those of morphine, since a dissociation between ECoG and behavior became evident following morphine administration.

Some studies have also suggested that the environmental factors play an important role in determining the stimulating effects of morphine. This effect was absent in "experienced" mice (i.e., in subjects already tested in the apparatus), as compared with naive "inexperienced" animals.

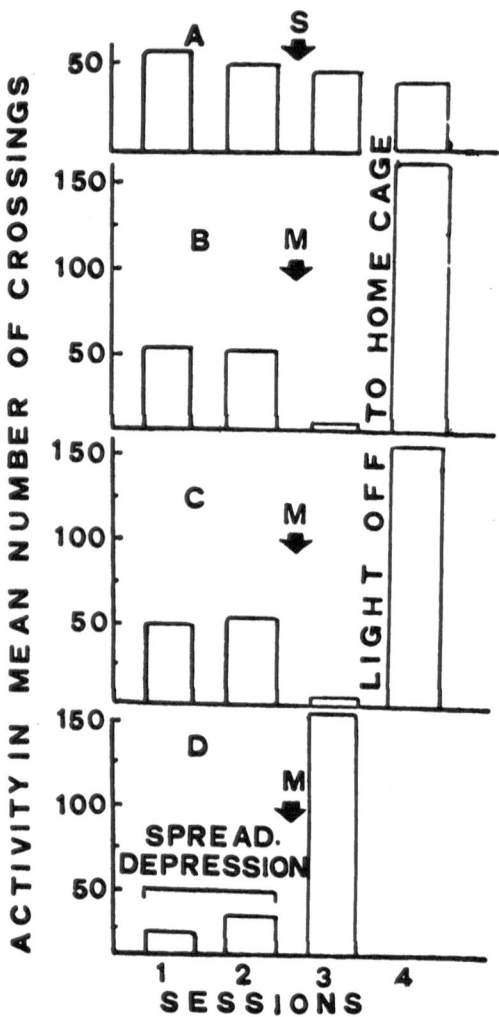

**Figure 4.** Effects of past experience on the morphine-induced "running fit." Groups A and D were subjected to two 25-min-long sessions (1 and 2), spaced by 6 hours. Animals of group D were subjected to cortical spreading depression during these two sessions. Immediately after the session, two of the mice were injected with 20 mg/kg of saline (S) or morphine (M) and tested again for 25 min (session 3). At the end of this session, the mice were either returned to their home cage for 2 to 3 minutes and then tested again for 25 minutes (session 4), or they were subjected to an additional session in total darkness. The performance of groups A and B during the third and fourth sessions was significantly different (t = 13.1, P <0.001; t = 17.0, P < 0.001). Similarly, the performance of group C during session 4 was different from that of a control group (not shown) injected with saline and subjected to a similar schedule (t = 14.9, P<0.001). In the mice tested under spreading depression during sessions 1 and 2, morphine significantly enhanced the performance in relation to that of another group of animals injected with saline (t = 17.9, P < 0.001) (Oliverio and Castellano, 1974a).

# H. REFERENCES

Alleva, E., Castellano, C., and Oliverio, A. (1980). Effects of L- and D-Aminoacids on analgesia and locomotor activity of mice. Their interaction with morphine. *Brain Res.* 198:249-252.

Bläsig, J., Herz, A., Reinhold, K., and Zieglgänsberger, S. (1973). Development of physical dependence on morphine in respect to time and dosage and quantification of the precipitated withdrawal syndrome in rats. *Psychopharmacologia.* 33:19-38.

Bovet, D., Bovet-Nitti, F., and Oliverio, A. (1969). Genetic aspects of learning and memory in mice. *Sci.* 163:139-149.

Bovet, D., Bovet-Nitti, F., and Oliverio, A. (1966). Action of nicotine on spontaneous and acquired behavior in rats and mice. *Ann. N.Y. Acad. Sci.* 142:261-267.

Brown, A.M. (1959). The investigation of specific responses in laboratory animals. Symposium. Laboratory Animals Centre, Royal Veterinary College, London pp. 9-16.

Buxbaum, D.M., Yarbrough, G.G., and Carter, M.E. (1973). Biogenic amines and narcotic effects. I. Modification of morphine-induced analgesia and motor activity after alteration of cerebral amine levels. *J. Pharmacol. Exp. Ther.* 185:317-327.

Castellano, C., and Oliverio, A. (1975). A genetic analysis of morphine induced running and analgesia in the mouse. *Psychopharmacologia.* 41:197-200.

Castellano, C., Espinet Llovera, B., and Oliverio, A. (1975). Morphine induced running and analgesia in two strains of mice following septal lessions or modification of brain amines. *Arch. Pharmacol.* 288:355-370.

Castellano, C., Filibeck, U., and Oliverio, A. (1976). Effects of heroin, alone or in combination with other drugs, on the locomotor activity in two inbred strains of mice. *Psychopharmacologia.* 49:29-31.

Cheney, D.L., and Goldstein, A. (1971). The effect of p-Chlorophenylalanine on opiate-induced running, analgesia, tolerance, and physical dependence in mice. *J. Pharmacol. Exp. Ther.* 177:309-315.

Cochin, J., and Kornetsky, C. (1964). Development and loss of tolerance to morphine in rats after single and multiple injection. *J. Pharmacol. Exp. Ther.* 145:1-10.

Cox, B.M., Ginsburg, M. and Osman, O.H. (1968). Acute tolerance to narcotic analgesic drugs in rats. *Brit. J. Pharmacol.* 33:245-256.

Criswell, E.H., and Levitt, R.A. (1975). The narcotic analgesics, in *Psychopharmacology: A Biological Approach.* R.A. Levitt, ed. John Wiley and Sons, New York. pp. 187-230.

Domino, E.F., and Wilson, A. (1973). Effects of narcotic analgesic agonists and antagonists on rat brain acetylcholine. *J. Pharmacol. Exp. Ther.* 184:18-32.

Ebel, A., Hermetet, J.C., and Mandel, P. (1973). Comparative study of acetylcholinesterase and choline-acetyltransferase enzyme activity in brain of DBA and C57 mice. *Nat. New Biol.* 242:56-57.

Eddy, N.B., and Leimback, D. (1953). Synthetic analgesics. II. Dithienylbutenyl-and dithienyl-butylamines. *J. Pharmacol. Exp. Ther.* 107:385-393.

Eleftheriou, B.E. (1971). Regional brain norepinephrine turnover rates in four strains of mice. *Neuroendocrinol.* 7:329-336.

Elias, M.F. (1970). Differences in reversal learning between two inbred mouse strains. *Psychonom. Sci.* 20:179-180.

Eriksson, K. (1969). Factors affecting voluntary alcohol consumption in the albino rat. *Ann. Zool. Fenn.* 6:227-236.

Eriksson, K., and Kiianmaa, K. (1971). Genetic analysis of susceptibility to morphine addiction in inbred mice. *Ann. Med. Exp. Fenn.* 49:73-78.

Evangelista, A.M., Gattoni, R.C., and Izquierdo, I. (1970). Effects of amphetamine, nicotine, and hexamethonium on performance of a conditioned response during acquisition and retention trails. *Pharmacol.* 3:91-96.

Fuller, J.L. (1970). Strain differences in the effects of chlorpromazine and chlordiazepoxide upon active and passive avoidance in mice. *Psychopharmacologia* 16:261–271.

Fuller, J.L. (1966). Variation of effects of chlorpromazine in three strains of mice. *Psychopharmacologia.* 8:408–414.

Fuller, J.L. (1964). Measurement of alcohol preference in genetic experiments. *J. Comp. Physiol. Psychol.* 57:85–88.

Gebhart, G.F., and Mitchell, C.L. (1973). Strain differences in the analgesic response to morphine as measured on the hot-plat. *Arch. Int. Pharmacodyn. Thér.* 201:128–135.

Giarman, N.J., and Pepeu, G. (1962). Drug induced changes in brain acetylcholine. *Brit. J. Pharmacol.* 19:226–234.

Gillette, J.R. (1965). Drug toxicity as a result of interference with physiological mechanisms. *Ann. N.Y. Acad. Sci.* 123:42–53.

Goldstein, A., and Sheehan, P. (1969). Tolerance to opioid narcotics. I. Tolerance to the "running fit" caused by Levorphanol in the mouse. *J. Pharmacol. Exp. Ther.* 169:175–184.

Herz, A., Albus, K., Metys, J., Schubert, P., and Teschemaker, H. (1970). On the central sites for the antinociceptive action of morphine and fentanyl. *Neuropharmacol.* 9:539–551.

Herz, A., Bläsig, J., and Papeschi, R. (1974). Role of catecholaminergic mechanisms in the expression of the morphine abstinence syndrome in rats. *Psychopharmacologia.* 39:121–143.

Hollinger, M. (1969). Effects of reserpine, $\alpha$-methyl-p-tyrosine, p-chlorophenylalanine, and pargyline on levorphanol induced running activity in mice. *Arch. Int. Pharmacodyn Thér.* 179:419–424.

Huidobro, J.P., and Huidobro, F. (1973). Acute morphine tolerance in new born and young rats. *Psychopharmacologia.* 28:27–34.

Jhamandas, K., and Dickinson, G. (1973). Modification of precipitated morphine and methadone abstinence by acetylcholine antagonists. *Nat. New Biol.* 245:219–221.

Jhamandas, K., Pinsky, C., and Phillis, J.W. (1970). Effects of morphine and its antagonists on release of cerebral cortical acetylcholine. *Nat.* 238:176–177.

Kalow, K. (1966). Genetic aspects of drug safety. *App. Ther.* 8:44–46.

Kempf, E., Greilsamer, J., Mack, G., and Mandel, P. (1974). Correlation of behavioral differences in three strains of mice with differences in brain amines. *Nat.* 247:483–485.

Koppanyi, T., and Avery, M.A. (1966). Species differences and the clinical trial of new drugs: A review. *Clin. Pharmacol. Ther.* 7:250–254.

Kuhar, M.J., Pert, B.C., and Snyder, S.H. (1973). Regional distribution of opiate receptor binding in monkey and human brain. *Nat.* 245:447–450.

Laschka, E., Teschemaker, H., Mehrain, P., and Herz, A. (1976). Sites of action of morphine involved in the development of physical dependence in rats. *Psychopharmacologia.* 46:141–147.

Lindzey, G., Loehlin, J., Manosevitz, M., and Thiessen, D.D. (1971). Behavioral genetics. *Ann. Rev. Psychol.* 22:39–94.

Lotti, J.V., Lomax, P., and George, R. (1966). Acute tolerance to morphine following systemic and intracerebral injection in the rat. *Int. J. Neuropharmacol.* 5:32–42.

Mack, C., Greilsamer, J., Kempf, E., and Mandel, P. (1973). Neurochemical correlates of genetically observed differences in performance levels in mice. Abstract IV. Int. Meeting of the International Society of Neurochemistry, Tokyo.

Mandel, P., Ebel, A., Hermetet, J.C., Bovet, D., and Oliverio, A. (1973). Etudes des enzymes du système cholinergique chez les hybrides $F_1$ de souris se distinguant par leur aptitude au conditionnement. *C.R. Acad. Sci.* 276:395–398.

McClearn, G.E., and Rodgers, D.A. (1959). Differences in alcohol preference among inbred strains of mice. *Quart. J. Stud. Alc.* 20:691–695.

McClearn, G.E., Wilson, J.R., and Meredith, W. (1970). The use of isogenic and heterogenic mouse stocks in behavioral research, in *Contributions to Behavior-Genetic Analysis: The Mouse as a Prototype.* G. Lindzey and D.D. Thiessen, eds. Appleton-Century-Crofts, New York.

Meier, H. (1963). Factors influencing drug metabolism, in *Experimental Pharmacogenetics.* Academic Press, New York. pp. 9-75.

Oliverio, A. (1975). Genotype dependent electroencephalographic behavioral and analgesic correlates of morphine: An analysis in normal mice and in mice with septal lesions. *Brain Res.* 83:135-141.

Oliverio, A. (1968). Neurohumoral systems and learning, in *Psychopharmacology, a Review of Progress, 1957-1967.* Public Health Service Publication D.H. Efron, ed. Washington, D.C. No. 1936, pp. 867-868.

Oliverio, A., and Castellano, C. (1974a). Experience modifies morphine induced behavioral excitation of mice. *Nat.* 252:229-230.

Oliverio, A., and Castellano, C. (1974b). Genotype-dependent sensitivity and tolerance to morphine and heroin: Dissociation between opiate-induced running and analgesia in the mouse. *Psychopharmacologia.* 39:13-22.

Oliverio, A., and Castellano, C. (1973). Pharmacogenetic aspects of learning and memory, in *Proceedings Fifth International Congress of Pharmacology, San Francisco, 1972.* G.H. Acheson, F.E. Bloom, J. Cochin, T.A. Loomis, R.A. Maxwell, and G.T. Okita, eds. Karger, Basel.

Oliverio, A., Castellano, C., and Messeri, P. (1973). Genotype dependent effects of septal lesions on different types of learning in the mouse. *J. Comp. Physiol. Psychol.* 82:240-246.

Pepeu, G., Mulas, A. Ruffi, A., and Sotgiu, P. (1971). Brain acetylcholine levels in rats with septal lesions. *Life Sci.* 10:181-184.

Pert, C.B., and Snyder, S.H. (1973). Opiate receptor: Demonstration in nervous tissue. *Sci.* 179:1011-1014.

Quinn, G., Axelrod, J., and Brodie, B.B. (1954). Species and sex differences in metabolism and duration of hexobarbital. *Fed. Proc.* 13:395.

Reggiani, A., Battaini, F., Kobayashi, H., Spans, P.F., and Trabucchi, M. (1980). Genotype-dependent sensitivity to morphine: role of different receptor populations. *Brain Res.* 189:289-294.

Renzi, P., and Sansone, M. (1971). Discriminated lever-press avoidance in mice. *Comm. Behav. Biol.* 6:315-321.

Rethy, C.R., Smith, C.B., and Villarreal, J.E. (1971). Effects of narcotic analgesics upon the locomotor activity and brain catecholamine content of the mouse. *J. Pharmacol. Exp. Ther.* 176:472-479.

Samanin, R., and Valzelli, L. (1972). Serotoninergic neurotransmission and morphine activity. *Arch. Int. Pharmacodyn. Thér.* 196:138-141.

Sansone, M., and Messeri, P. (1973). Strain differences in the effects of chlordiazepoxide and chlorpromazine on avoidance behavior of mice. *Pharmacol. Res. Comm.* 6:179-185.

Schlesinger, K., and Griek, B.J. (1970). The genetics and biochemistry of audiogenic seizures, in *Contributions to Behaviorgenetic Analysis: The Mouse as a Prototype.* G. Lindzey and D.D. Thiessen, eds. Appleton-Century-Crofts, New York. p. 219.

Seevers, M.H., and Deneau, G.A. (1963). Physiological aspects of tolerance and physical dependence, in *Physiological Pharmacology.* W.S. Root and F.G. Hofmann, eds. Academic Press, New York. Vol. 1, pp. 565-640.

Sharkawi, M. (1970). Effects of morphine and pentobarbitone on acetylcholine synthesis by rat cerebral cortex. *Brit. J. Pharmacol.* 40:86-91.

Shuster, L., Hannam, R.V., and Boyle, W.E., Jr. (1963). A simple method for producing tolerance to dihydromorphinone in mice. *J. Pharmacol. Exp. Ther.* 140:149-154.

Sprott, R.L. (1971). Inheritance of avoidance learning. *Jackson Lab. Ann. Rep.* 42:78-85.

Srebro, B., Oderfeld-Novak, B., Klodos, I., Dabrowka, J., and Narkiewicz, O. (1973). Changes in acetylcholinesterase activity in hippocampus produced by septal lesions in the rat. *Life Sci.* 12:261-270.

Staats, J.L. (1972). Standard nomenclature for inbred strains of mice: Fifth listing. *Cancer Res.* 32:1609-1630.

Trabucchi, M., Spano, P.F., Racagni, G., and Oliverio, A (1976). Genotype-dependent sensitivity to morphine: Dopamine involvement in morphine-induced running in the mouse. *Brain Res.* 14:536-540.

Valatx, J.L., Bugat, R., and Jouvet, M. (1972). Genetic studies of sleep in mice. *Nat.* 238:226-227.

van Abeelen, J.H.F. (1966). Effects of genotype on mouse behaviour. *Anim. Behav.* 14:218-220.

Villarreal, J.E., Guzman, M., and Smith, C.B. (1973). A comparison of the effects of d-amphetamine and morphine upon the locomotor activity of mice treated with drugs which alter brain catecholamine content. *J. Pharmacol. Exp. Ther.* 187:1-7.

Wahlsten, D. (1972). Genetic experiments with animal learning: A critical review. *Behav. Biol.* 7:143-182.

Way, E.L., Ho, I.K., and Loh, H.H. (1973). Relations of brain serotonin to the inhibition and enhancement of morphine tolerance and physical dependence, in *New Concepts in Neurotransmitter Regulation*. A.J. Mandell, ed. Plenum Press, New York.

Wey, E., Loh, H.H., and Way, E.L. (1973). Brain sites of precipitated abstinence in morphine-dependent rats. *J. Pharmacol. Exp. Ther.* 185:108-115.

Williams, R.T. (1962). *Altered Drug Metabolism*. Ciba Foundation Symposium on Enzymes and Drug Action. Little, Brown & Co., Boston. pp. 239-244.

Wimer, C.C., Wimer, R.E., and Roderick. T.H. (1971). Some behavioral differences associated with relative size of hippocampus in the mouse. *J. Comp. Physiol. Psychol.* 76:57-65.

Yarbrough, G.G., Buxbaum, D.M., and Sanders-Bush, E. (1973). Biogenic amines and narcotic effects. II. Serotonin turnover in the rat after acute and chronic morphine administration. *J. Pharmacol. Exp. Ther.* 185:328-335.

Current Developments in Psychopharmacology, Volume 6
© 1981, Spectrum Publications, Inc.

CHAPTER 3

# ANTICONVULSANT DRUGS, BEHAVIOR, AND COGNITIVE ABILITIES

## MICHAEL TRIMBLE

The literature concerning the relationship of anticonvulsant drugs to disturbances of behavior and cognitive abilities has been reviewed. It is indicated that although completed studies are sparse and although many of the techniques currently used for evaluating the effects of such drugs on patients are inadequate, certain conclusions may be drawn. With regard to the effects on cognitive abilities, the drugs not only impair performance on psychological tests, but some drugs—particularly phenytoin—are associated with a progressive decline of intellectual abilities, which is often insidious and unrecognized. There is little systematic evidence to indicate which anticonvulsant drugs have adverse effects on behavior, but several studies have indicated improvements in behavior associated with carbamazepine and sulthiame.

The possible reasons why anticonvulsant drugs should have these effects are discussed, and particularly the relationship of the drugs to abnormal folic acid and monoamine metabolism are highlighted.

## A. INTRODUCTION

Although many authors have commented on changes in behavior associated with anticonvulsant drugs, the type of behavior referred to is often not clearly specified. In this review, the effects that these drugs have on cognitive function have been separated from other effects on behavior on the grounds that such an initial separation leads to a better understanding of the situation and provides a better basis for future studies.

## B. DRUGS AND COGNITIVE BEHAVIOR

Deterioration of the mental state in epilepsy has been commented on since antiquity. Tempkin (1971) quotes Aretaeus as saying that epileptics were "languid, spiritless, stupid, unsociable . . . [and] slow to learn from torpidity of the understanding and the senses." Nearer to the present time, Gowers (1885) comments, "The mental state of epileptics frequently presents deterioration. . . . In its slighter forms there is merely defective memory . . . in more severe degree there is greater imperfection of intellectual power."

Upholding the view that seems to have been predominant in the latter part of the last century, he attributed this deterioration to the underlying epilepsy. Other authors supported this view, quoting, for example, studies that showed institutionalized epileptics as having low IQ's (Fox, 1924). However, a distinct paradox remains. History has many examples of highly intelligent epileptics who did not deteriorate with their illness—Pliny, Caligula, Petrarch, Caesar, Napoleon, and Handel, to name but a few.

Guerrant et al. (1962) have reviewed the changing concepts of the nature and frequency of mental changes in epileptics in the last century, culminating in the present view that the majority of patients have normal mental states; and in those in whom deterioration occurs, many different factors may operate, although the relative importance of each of these is still a matter of uncertainty and disagreement. Guerrant et al. comment that a minority of authors have occasionally implicated a deleterious effect of anticonvulsant drugs, but generally this has been doubted, apart from well-recognized sedative effects, and not submitted to investigation. More recently, with increasing recognition of some of the chronic metabolic and structural effects of anticonvulsant therapy (Reynolds, 1975a), and the development of techniques for measuring serum anticonvulsant levels (Woodbury et al., 1972), more serious attention has been directed at the possible role of such therapy in the deterioration of the mental state.

The studies of Lennox (1942) represent the first systematic attempt to investigate the role that anticonvulsants play in mental deterioration. In a paper entitled "Brain Injury, Drugs and Environment as Causes of Mental Decay in Epilepsy," he tried to assess what drugs had been used in a series of 1245 epileptic patients, and what effects these drugs had on their seizures and mental state. He examined five possible causes for mental deterioration: (1) heredity; (2) brain injury antedating the onset of seizures; (3) psychological handicaps; (4) epilepsy itself; and finally (5) drugs. He estimated that anticonvulsant drugs were incriminated in this process in 15 percent of his cases, and commented that "many physicians in attempting to extinguish seizures only succeed in drowning the finer intellectual processes of their patients. . . . The intelligent and individualistic use of anticonvulsant drugs should not and does not impair the patient's mind." At the time Lennox undertook his study, bromides, phenobarbitone, and a variety of proprietary remedies were the only drugs available for the treatment of epilepsy, and his findings indicated that phenobarbitone was the most effective anticonvulsant, and that it impaired mental processes the least.

Writing on the same subject 18 years later, Lennox still implicated the same five causes, but now held that anticonvulsants were only responsible for approximately 5 percent of the cases of mental deterioration that he encountered (Lennox and Lennox, 1960).

In view of these observations, and with the introduction of phenytoin in 1938 and subsequently a succession of other anticonvulsant drugs, many studies of drug effects on mental processes might have been expected. However, while the acute effects of the new drugs were soon noted and recorded, chronic toxic side effects, especially with regard to mental changes, seem to have received scant attention. The data that have been collected are reviewed below taking as far as possible individual drugs separately.

In retrospect, it does not seem unlikely that such mental effects may occur. Epilepsy, more often than not, is a lifelong disorder. It requires continuous medication over a considerable number of years, and treatment is often initiated in the early years of life and hence may influence a developing nervous system.

## 1. Studies of Individual Drugs

### a. Bromides

At one time, the main therapy for epilepsy was bromides. In recent years, these drugs have ceased to be of clinical importance and therefore will not be discussed. That these drugs were capable of adversely affecting the mental state is illustrated by the fact that bromism accounted for 4 percent of admissions to psychopathic hospitals in the early part of this century (Merritt, 1955).

### b. Phenobarbitone

In the 1920s and 1930s, the prevalent view was that phenobarbitone had no adverse effect on mental function, other than its soporific action, as is emphasised, for example, in the clinical reports of Grinker (1929) and Barnes and Fetterman (1938).

Lennox (1942) assessed the effects of anticonvulsants on mentality and reported that while 30 percent of 638 patients examined on phenobarbitone improved, 58 percent were unchanged and 12 percent worsened. This was marginally better than the bromides and considerably better than "patent drugs."

A controlled trial by Somerfeld-Ziskind and Ziskind (1940) in 100 patients included a battery of 6 psychological tests. Although the control population of this study is inadequate and the statistics are sparse, they state with confidence "This study indicates that phenobarbital in doses of 0.1 g two or three times a day can be given without resultant deterioration of intellect."

Wapner et al. (1962) examined 36 epileptic children between the ages of 8 and 12. They assessed their intelligence and learning abilities before and after 6 weeks of treatment with phenobarbitone. To rule out learning effects, they did the same tests on a control group of matched normal children. They tested vocabulary acquisition and T-style maze performance. They found no statistical difference in the performance of the epileptic children at the two test periods; however, they report that initial preformance on a T-stylus maze was superior in the control group, but the net gain in the two groups in this index during the period of the trial was in fact the same.

In contrast with these negative findings, in a psychometric study of 20 epileptics, Tchicaloff and Gaillard (1970) found a correlation between dose of phenobarbitone and impaired performance on some subtests of the W.A.I.S. They clearly implicate the drug as responsible for this deterioration.

A 1-month study by Hutt et al. (1968) on normal adults also suggested that phenobarbitone impairs performance in certain psychological tests of perceptual-motor behavior, i.e. key pressing, vigilance, verbal learning, and speech rate. These results will be discussed later in the section on anticonvulsant drug levels.

### c. Phenytoin

Many of the early clinical reports following the introduction of phenytoin in 1938 suggested a positive psychotropic effect of the drug leading to improved alertness. It seems likely that such effects resulted from improved seizure control and reduction of previously heavy doses of phenobarbitone or bromides.

It was soon recognized that acute toxic doses of phenytoin had adverse effects on the mental states of epileptics, leading to a confusional state— sometimes referred to as encephalopathy—associated with neurological signs of toxicity, especially nystagmus and ataxia. The early literature is reviewed by Finkelman and Arieff (1942), who described four cases of their own, and the whole syndrome has been well reviewed by Roseman (1961).

He reported on the association of such symptoms as ataxia, nystagmus, etc., with such behavioral abnormalities as depression, drowsiness, and even euphoria. In this "toxic" state, there were accompanying electroencephalographic (EEG) changes of alpha-slowing with the appearance of delta waves. Later studies on similar patients with "pseudodegenerative" presentations using serum level measurements indicate that they were related to unrecognized toxicity with phenytoin.

In relation to possible chronic effects on psychological function, Booker et al. (1967) employed a battery of psychological tests in a controlled study in 17 normal students who were given 100 mg of phenytoin 3 times daily, or a placebo for 6 days. No consistent effects attributable to the drug were found.

Rosen (1968) commented that decreased intellectual performance may be a complication of long-term phenytoin therapy in some epileptics in view of his observations in 20 such patients in whom school work performance improved rapidly when the drug was discontinued for various reasons. The improvement was associated with corresponding changes in W.A.I.S., Bender-Gestalt, and other tests of intellectual and perceptual performance, but few details were given. A similar finding was reported by Vallarta et al. (1974). They observed 10 patients with progressive neurological deterioration and impaired intellectual performance, which they attributed directly to an effect of the drug. The deterioration stopped when the drug was removed, but in only six of the children was their pretherapy condition restored.

In a more recent study of the effects of a variety of factors associated with the performance and progress of epileptic children attending ordinary schools, it was found that children who were on phenytoin for at least 2 years had significantly inferior reading skills when compared to children on other anticonvulsants (Stores, 1975), lending support to Rosen's observations.

Other studies with this drug have been undertaken since the introduction of measurement of serum levels of anticonvulsants. These are described below.

### d. Ethosuximide

Using a test/retest situation, the effects of this drug were assessed in 25 children with petit mal epilepsy by Guey et al. (1967). At the start of the experiment, the children were receiving other anticonvulsants, which were continued. The children were then reassessed after a period of several months on ethosuximide. The authors claimed that this drug caused psychic disturbance that affected both the intellectual and affective spheres, the former mainly showing as memory and speech disturbances. These effects were seen most markedly in older patients and in those who were receiving higher doses of the drug. This study, however, must be interpreted with caution for several reasons: (1) 15 of their 25 patients were mentally retarded; (2) the patients were receiving other drugs at the time of the trial; (3) they did not include a control group for comparison. The importance of proper controls in such a study as this is paramount, especially as it has been shown that EEG spike-wave activity of petit mal epilepsy may be correlated with impaired visual-motor performance (Goode et al., 1970).

An important feature that the study reemphasizes, however, is the necessity to explore as many individual components of intellectual functioning as possible. Thus, if an overall assessment is taken, such as full-scale IQ, verbal IQ, or performance IQ, significant difference may not be—and in fact were not—obtained. More subtle subtests, however, may yield significant results; and in this investigation the subtests in which significant differences emerged were comprehension, memory, and spatiotemporal perceptual difficulties. In a more extended study of 100 patients with petit mal epilepsy receiving ethosuximide, Soulayrol and Roger (1970) confirmed their earlier findings and concluded that intellectual efficiency falls significantly in most of the children treated with the drug.

In a study on children with learning disorders and 14–6 positive spike EEG patterns, Smith et al. (1968) found different results. The children under study had EEG abnormalities regarded as abnormal and indicative of cerebral dysfunction. Ten children were given ethosuximide or a placebo on a double-blind basis, and psychological testing was performed before and during ethosuximide administration. Significant increases were seen in verbal IQ scores, as measured on the WISC test between placebo and drug treatments, the mean difference being 12 points. No changes were observed on measures of performance or personality tests. They interpret this result as indicating that ethosuximide has some specific effect on the functions of the left hemisphere of the brain.

In a recent controlled study of 37 epileptic children with petit mal epilepsy, Browne et al. (1975) reported no deleterious effects of "therapeutic" blood levels of ethosuximide on psychometric performance over a period of 8 weeks. Furthermore, the performance of 17 of these patients improved; this was probably associated with the very good control of seizures achieved. They discuss several possible explanations for the discrepancy between their own findings and those of Guey et al. (1967). These include different length of follow-up; different populations under study, in that in the study of Browne et al. fewer patients were retarded; and a different age of the two populations, those in Guey's group containing more adolescents.

### e. Carbamazepine

This drug, developed in the early 1950s, was first used in epilepsy in the 1960s. In the original study on the drug in epileptic patients, Bonduelle commented on the improvement in patients who had psychological disorders (Bonduelle et al., 1964). Since then it has been shown that the drug is effective in the management of a variety of epileptic disorders, and there are multiple claims in the literature that it has psychotropic properties (see below).

Schain et al. (1977) evaluated the results of changing children with epilepsy from their conventional anticonvulsant onto carbamazepine. They administered a battery of psychological tests including the WISC, Matched Familiar Figures test, and the Porteus Maze. Highly significant differences were found on all the tests used, and in particular they note "substantial improvement on all measures dependent on cognitive styles facilitating problem solving." Change in seizure frequency was not related to this improvement. Unfortunately, they could not, with the design of this trial, eliminate practice effects. In that the experiment was designed to take children off "sedative" anticonvulsants, the study prompts the question as to whether the improvements noted were due to stopping the initial drugs, or to a direct effect of the carbamazepine, a question first raised shortly after the introduction of carbamazepine (Parsonage, 1975).

Rett (1976) conducted a similar study on 10 patients with grand mal epilepsy (aged 13 to 16), changing them from their existing drugs to carbamazepine and retesting on a variety of psychological tests (including the WISC) 11 to 12 months later. No significant changes were noted, although assessment of verbal IQ showed a mean increase of 7 points, and overall IQ a mean increase of 5 points. The difference between this result and that of Schain et al. (1977) may be due to the small number of children used and thus the absence of "statistically significant" detectable results. Rett also gave 10 other epileptic patients, who were not on anticonvulsants, carbamazepine and assessed pretreatment/posttreatment scores. Estimations of motor function (the Walther Test was used, which the authors felt was "probably the most suitable test of psychomotor function") showed significant improvements in the carbamazepine-treated group.

The drug has also been used in the management of a variety of behavior disorders in childhood, and some studies have thus been carried out on nonepileptic children. Although favorable effects of carbamazepine on psychological tests have been indicated, the trials are uncontrolled and often reported without a full presentation of the data and relevant statistics (Krasovsky et al., 1972; de Weis et al., 1974).

One double-blind controlled trial of crossover design in 20 children with behavior disorders did demonstrate improvement in performance on measures of concentration, but it is unclear whether the improvement was a consequence of the improved behavior disorder that was also found (Groh et al., 1971). In a double-blind comparison between the effects of adding primidone or carbamazepine to patients already receiving phenytoin at a therapeutic level, it has been shown that primidone resulted in a greater impairment of cognitive function, especially on a perceptual-motor battery than did carbamazepine. However, full results were not given (Rodin et al., 1976).

### f. Other Anticonvulsants

Information regarding the effect of other anticonvulsants, some of them widely used in the management of epilepsy, is sparse. Hutt, et al. (1966) have investigated the effect of sulthiame on the attention span of a hyperkinetic child and shown that it increased the span in both small (50 mg t.i.d.) and large doses (100 mg q.i.d.). Green et al. (1974), however, report that patients on sulthiame do not perform as well as when on phenytoin on the modified Reitan battery, although details of the results are not given. Dodrill (1975b) recently compared the effects of sulthiame with phenytoin on a variety of neuropsychological tests. Twenty-two epileptic patients were given either phenytoin or sulthiame in a double-blind fashion, after a 2-month stabilization period on phenytoin. Measurements included WAIS; Halstead Neuropsychological battery; Trail-Making test, and a series of tests of perceptual function. The patients were also given a rating scale of social functioning. All subtests of the WAIS favored phenytoin, and many differences reached statistical significance, especially on verbal scores. Similar results in favor of phenytoin were recorded on other tests, which the authors felt were an indication of concentration and sustained attention to task. On the social-functioning scale, results with phenytoin were significantly different from sulthiame on work and finance and on the total positive score. While these results are clear, unfortunately many patients did not complete the study and the tested patients were thus a baised sample. Additionally, many more seizures occurred in the patients on sulthiame, a factor which may itself interfere with performance.

Although widely used in the management of epilepsy, there do not seem to be any data available with regard to the effects of primidone on performance, although toxic effects due to the primidone are suspected (Booker, 1972). One study has suggested that this drug may be implicated in a deteriorative effect on cognitive function similar to that of phenytoin (Trimble et al., 1978b). Few data are available with respect to sodium valproate, apart from some uncontrolled trials, which suggest that it may improve visuomotor coordination (Schlack, 1974), and improve alertness and school performance (Barnes and Bower, 1975). Recently, it has been reported as hypnotic in normal volunteers, an effect enhanced by the simultaneous administration of phenobarbitone (Boxer et al., 1976).

### 2. Studies Not Separating Drugs

Loveland et al. (1975), in an extensive study of 26 epileptic patients on anticonvulsant drugs, assessed their psychological abilities over a period of 3 months in a test/retest situation. From a battery of psychometric tests, they were able to derive 2000 separate items on which statistical analyses were possible. Only 44 of these were significant, and the general conclusion of the authors was that the drugs administered had little or no effect on the patients' total adjustment to their environment. However, there was no control for the dose of the various drugs given. Furthermore, the majority of the patients were already receiving their anticonvulsants for some years prior to the study, and it is perhaps not surprising that no decline in performance was seen over a subsequent 3-month period. Only five patients were not on medication at the initial testing. When retested, this group improved less in their delayed recall than in their matched controls.

Royo and Martin (1959) described three epileptic children who were given full psychological testing while receiving anticonvulsant therapy with multiple drugs. They suggested that anticonvulsants not only lower intellectual efficiency in general, but have a particularly impressive effect on visuo-perceptive and visuo-spatial discrimination. These effects they considered to be due to "ill-balanced therapy."

Tchicaloff and Gaillard (1970) reported that phenobarbitone and phenytoin together do impair mental function; and on tests of visuo-spatial performance, significant cumulative effects of the drugs were observable. Kerfriden (1970) supported their conclusions and stated that anticonvulsant medication seems to be an obstacle to learning in the epileptic child.

In contrast, in their controlled study of 28 epileptic children who showed intellectual deterioration (as measured by decline in IQ scores), Chaudhry and Pond (1961) found no evidence to implicate anticonvulsants as a cause for this and suggested that the deterioration was related to seizure frequency. However, drug intake was assessed using a rating scale which assumed that 60 mg of phenobarbitone was equivalent to 100 mg of phenytoin and 0.5 g of primidone.

In a study of 117 epileptic children at ordinary schools, Holdsworth and Whitmore (1974) found no difference in educational outcome according to whether or not phenobarbitone was being prescribed. No indication is given of the dosages employed or what other drugs were being taken. Educational performance was assessed on questionnaires completed from interviews with teachers, without specific testing of the children.

## 3.  Studies Including Serum Anticonvulsant levels

The development of techniques for the measurement of serum anticonvulsant levels has been a significant factor in stimulating interest in the effects of anticonvulsants on mental processes. Conventionally, the drugs have been administered by increasing the dose until seizures are controlled, or until toxic signs are produced, when the dose is marginally reduced. The first sign of toxicity is usually thought to be nystagmus, and some have even considered it desirable that nystagmus should be present in a patient receiving anticonvulsant medication (Haerer and Grace, 1969). With the ability to detect anticonvulsants in the serum, "therapeutic" and "toxic" levels have recently been defined for several anticonvulsants (Woodbury et al., 1972).

It is now apparent that intoxication is better correlated with serum level than with daily dosage. Kutt et al. (1964) reported a close correlation between individual signs of toxicity and serum levels of phenytoin, with mental confusion occurring only above $160 \mu$ mol/l. Other evidence, however, does not reveal such a precise relationship. Individual variation is apparent and not all patients exhibit the classical signs to toxicity (Reynolds, 1970).

### a. Subacute or Chronic Phenytoin Encephalopathy

Although a confusional state, sometimes referred to as encephalopathy, delirium, or psychosis, has long been recognized as an acute toxic effect of phenytoin associated with other clear neurological evidence of toxicity, such as nystagmus and ataxia (Finkelman and Arieff, 1942; Kutt et al., 1964; Glaser, 1972), the measurement of serum levels of the drug has recently revealed that a subacute or chronic reversible impairment of intellectual function, awareness, and mood due to the drug may easily be overlooked due to the absence of the classical signs of toxicity.

Husby (1963) who measured serial blood levels of the drug in 151 patients over a period of 5 to 18 months, noted the insidious development of depression in 3 and dementia in 2 associated with serum concentrations between 136 and $232 \mu$ mol/l. Some had mild disturbance of gait, but nystagmus was not recorded, and the mental symptoms disappeared on reduction of therapy. Frantzen et al. (1967) and Reynolds (1970) also noted a much broader variety of psychiatric and neurological complications of insidious phenytoin toxicity as a result of serum level measurements. Intellectual deterioration, depression, and aggravation of behavior disorders were included in the spectrum encountered. Impairment of drive and initiative, psychomotor slowing, and lowering of mood were particularly common (Reynolds, 1970).

Examples of this encephalopathy have been stressed, particularly in children in whom nystagmus and ataxia may not occur, especially in the presence of pre-existing brain damage or mental retardation, and in whom further deterioration in intellectual function may be overlooked, or mistakenly regarded as part of an underlying progressive neurological disease that may be responsible for the fits (Patel and Crichton, 1968; Rosen, 1968; Logan and Freeman, 1969; Weiss et al., 1969; Prensky et al., 1971). Further examples in adults have been reported by Perlo and Schwab (1969) and Reynolds and Travers (1974). Sometimes the encephalopathy may be associated with unusual neurological signs, including involuntary movements (Kooiker and Sumi, 1974; McLellan and Swash, 1974), which may further perpetuate a vain search for underlying neurological disease. A modest rise of CSF protein may be found (Rawson, 1968). Although serum levels of the drug are nearly always in the toxic range, this syndrome may occasionally occur with "therapeutic" levels (Glaser, 1972; Ambrosetto et al., 1977).

The above evidence suggests that serious effects on mental function may occasionally occur with toxic levels of phenytoin in the absence of more classical signs of toxicity. Delay in recognition of such toxicity may result unless serum anticonvulsant levels are measured. Other more recent evidence suggests the possibility that mental symptoms, albeit of a more subtle kind, may be seen with blood levels below the generally recognized toxic range, especially if therapy is prolonged.

Reynolds and Travers (1974) studied a group of 57 outpatient epileptics on chronic therapy with phenytoin and phenobarbitone. Intellectual deterioration, psychiatric illness or personality change, and psychomotor slowing were recorded as present or absent on the basis of clinical assessment and (in 50 percent) psychometric studies. After excluding patients with overt drug toxicity, gross cerebral lesions, or mental symptoms preceding the onset of epilepsy, those with mental symptoms were found to have significantly higher concentrations of both phenobarbitone and phenytoin than patients without such mental changes (with the single exception of phenobarbitone in relation to psychomotor slowing, where the trend was similar but not statistically significant). That this was not merely a reflection of more frequent seizures, and hence higher dosage of drugs, was excluded when similar differences were noted in patients with infrequent seizures (less than one a month).

In the groups with mental changes, the mean serum levels of both phenytoin and phenobarbitone were within the range generally regarded as "therapeutic" (i.e., 40-80 $\mu$mol/l for phenytoin; 60-140 $\mu$mol/l for phenobarbitone), although a wide scatter was encountered. The implication was that in some patients, drug effects on mental processes may occur not only in the absence of physical signs of toxicity, but also with serum levels not generally regarded as toxic. They authors emphasized that considerable individual variation in tolerance to the mental effects of the drugs exists, and that apart from the level of the drug in the serum, the duration of therapy may be important.

Similar findings on a population of epileptic children at a hospital school have also been reported, where 312 children were examined neuropsychiatrically and estimates of their IQ function were made available (Trimble et al., 1978b). Significant negative correlations were found between phenytoin; phenobarbitone, and primidone anticonvulsant levels and measures of performance IQ. No such relationship was indicated for carbamazepine. In addition, a group of children whose IQ had fallen while at the school were identified. Their mean serum phenytoin and primidone levels were found to be significantly greater than the levels for the rest of the children. The serum levels of the children with deterioration of their IQ were within the so-called therapeutic range, and there was no relationship between this deterioration and the more conventional signs of anticonvulsant toxicity, such as nystagmus, etc. The levels for phenytoin were still significant when children with frequent seizures were omitted from the analysis, confirming the suggestion of Reynolds and Travers (1974) that the deteriorative effects were probably related to a drug effect. Phenobarbitone and carbamazepine did not seem implicated in this process.

Other evidence that mental effects may occur at relatively low or "therapeutic" levels is to be found in the studies of Hutt et al. (1968) and Ideström et al. (1972) in normal volunteers. In four normal adults treated with phenobarbitone for up to 1 month, the former authors found correlations between blood levels of the drug (which reached "therapeutic" levels) and impairment of various measures of perceptual-motor performance, including key-pressing, vigilance, verbal learning, and speech rate. Some tests, e.g., the Gibson Spiral Test, were impaired only at high levels (100 $\mu$mol/l) of the drug, but others, e.g., key-pressing and verbal learning, were increasingly impaired in proportion to the blood level. These findings reinforce the point that a broad spectrum of tests must be sampled before it can be said that a drug does *not* have significant effects, and that the difficulty and duration of the task as well as social constraints are important in assessing performance. For example, in a 30-minute test for vigilance, no deterioration was detected in the first 10 minutes, but thereafter decline in performance was rapid. Similar studies in larger numbers of subjects and in epileptic patients would seem to be indicated.

Ideström et al. (1972) administered only 3 doses of phenytoin to normal students, and at 24 hours found some correlation between blood levels of the drug, which were "subtherapeutic," and some measures or ratings of concentration and psychomotor performance, including reaction time and critical flicker fusion.

In assessing the difference in psychological performance between epileptic patients considered on serum levels of anticonvulsants to be "toxic" and "non-toxic," Matthews and Harley (1975) reported poorer mean test scores in the toxic group. There were 35 patients included under the definition "toxic," who had either phenobarbitone levels greater than 100 $\mu$mol/l, phenytoin levels greater than 76$\mu$mol/l, or primidone levels greater than 36 $\mu$mol/l. In addition to the WAIS, assessment included tests of both sensory discrimination and motor proficiency. The significant differences noted were in the Seashore Rhythm Test (requiring sustained auditory attention); the Knox Cube Test, which is a measure of immediate memory for a sequence of movements, and the Maze Co-ordination Test. The major differences were therefore in the tests of sustained concentration and attention span, memory, and on tests of motor coordination. The authors make the point that the levels they have used to assess "toxicity" are lower than the values usually accepted, providing further evidence that changes may occur at levels regarded as therapeutic.

Dodrill (1975a) has attempted to look more specifically at neuropsychological performance in epileptic patients measuring serum levels of phenytoin. Seventy adult patients were given neuropsychological tests that involved the Halstead-Reitan test battery, WAIS, and tests of motor coordination. The patients at the time of testing were on phenytoin alone, with other drugs being phased out prior to the experiment. They separated out the groups of patients, depending on whether the blood level was greater or less than $120\,\mu$mol/l. A number of significant differences were noted between the groups in tasks involving motor performance; and in general, the more complicated the motor task, the greater the difference.

The groups were controlled for age, education, and age of onset of seizures. Although the high-level group was having more seizures than the low-level group, this was not significant. In this study, all patients were examined clinically by a neurologist, and those with signs of toxicity were noted. When these were compared to non-toxic patients, it was found that while the levels were higher in them (mean $168.3\,\mu$mol/l, as compared to $98.8\,\mu$mol/l for the non-toxic), the significant differences on psychological tests were fewer, indicating that clinical examination alone was underestimating the psychological aspects of toxicity.

## 4. Comment

A summary of the main studies reviewed above is given in Table 1. It seems clear that anticonvulsant drugs do have some effect—generally deleterious—on cognitive abilities, but there have been relatively few studies conducted to explore the situation. The studies conducted have often (1) been uncontrolled, (2) used standardized techniques of assessment rather than using tests more specifically designed to detect drug effects, and (3) failed to take into account practice effects, IQ differences, etc.

The different effects of these drugs on cognitive function have been discussed. First, a toxic confusional state can occur, which is often an acute effect associated with other signs of toxicity. Secondly, there is a more direct effect on performance on psychological tests, mainly reflecting changes in concentration, motor behavior, and visuo-spatial abilities. The drugs most implicated in this effect seem to be phenytoin, sulthiame, and to a lesser extent phenobarbitone and primidone. Least implicated would seem to be

**Table 1. Summary of Studies of Psychological Function in Relation to Anticonvulsant Drugs**

| Author | Date | No. | Subjects | Control | Duration of Study | Drugs | Serum Levels | Effect on Mental State |
|---|---|---|---|---|---|---|---|---|
| Somerfeld-Ziskind and Ziskind | 1940 | 100 | Epileptics | Yes | 2 yr | Phenobarbitone | — | None |
| Loveland et al. | 1957 | 26 | Epileptics | Yes | 3 mo | Phenobarbitone Phenytoin Primidone | — | None |
| Royo and Martin | 1959 | 3 | Epileptics | No | Var. | Phenobarbitone Phenytoin Primidone Mesantoin | — | Impaired |
| Chaudhry and Pond | 1961 | 28 | Epileptics | Yes | — | Phenobarbitone Phenytoin Primidone | — | None |
| Wapner et al. | 1962 | 36 | Epileptics | Yes | 6 wk | Phenobarbitone | — | None |
| Booker et al. | 1967 | 17 | Normal | Yes | 6 da | Phenytoin | — | None |
| Guev et al. | 1967 | 25 | Epileptics | No | Av. 7 mo | Ethosuximide | — | Impaired |
| Smith et al. | 1968 | 10 | 14-6+ve | Yes | 3 wk | Ethosuximide | — | Improved |
| Hutt et al. | 1968 | 4 | Normal | Yes | 1 mo | Phenobarbitone | "Therapeutic" | Impaired |
| Rosen | 1968 | 20 | Epileptics | No | — | Phenytoin | — | Improved on withdrawing medication |

| Author | Year | N | Population | Controlled | Duration | Drug | Levels | Outcome |
|---|---|---|---|---|---|---|---|---|
| Tchicaloff and Gaillard | 1970 | 20 | Epileptics | No | — | Phenobarbitone Phenytoin | — | Impaired |
| Sculayrol and Roger | 1970 | 100 | Epileptics | No | — | Ethosuximide | — | Impaired |
| Ideström et al. | 1972 | 35 | Normal | No | 1 da | Phenytoin | "Subtherapeutic" | Impaired |
| Reynolds and Travers | 1974 | 57 | Epileptics | No | — | Phenobarbitone Phenytoin | "Therapeutic" | Impaired |
| Holdsworth and Whitmore | 1974 | 117 | Epileptics | No | — | Phenobarbitone Others not specified | — | None on educational outcome |
| Dodrill | 1975 | 22 | Epileptics | Yes | 6 mo | Phenytoin Sulthiame | — | Sulthiame worse than phenytoin |
| Browne et al. | 1975 | 37 | Epileptics | No | 8 wk | Ethosuximide | "Therapeutic" | No impairment Improved in 17 |
| Dodrill | 1975 | 70 | Epileptics | No | — | Phenytoin | High and low levels | Impairment greater with high levels |
| Rett | 1976 | 20 | Epileptics | No | 11–12 mo | Carbamazepine | — | Improvement on psychomotor tests |
| Schain et al. | 1977 | 45 | Epileptics | No | 4–6 mo | Carbamazepine | — | Improvement |
| Trimble et al. | 1978b | 312 | Epileptics | No | — | Carbamazepine Primidone Phenytoin Phenobarbitone | "Therapeutic" | Deterioration with phenytoin and primidone |

carbamazepine. Finally, there is a chronic deterioration of mental abilities that occurs mainly with phenytoin. It may occur at so-called "therapeutic" levels and is often unrecognized. Some patients, especially those with low IQ or brain damage, seem particularly susceptible to develop such a syndrome.

## C. THE EFFECTS OF ANTICONVULSANT DRUGS ON BEHAVIOR

There are even fewer studies on the effects of anticonvulsant drugs on behavior than on their effects on cognitive function. Again, many anecdotes are found in the literature but few attempts have been made to properly assess the situation.

Depression has been suggested as a side effect of phenobarbitone (Jeavons, 1975), phenytoin (Husby, 1963), sulthiame (Jeavons, 1975; Smyth, 1964), and peganone (Livingston, 1972). Personality changes have been recorded shortly after starting primidone (Booker, 1972). In addition, the occurrence of hysteria (Niedermeyer et al., 1970), hallucinations, delusions, and schizophreniform psychosis are reported in association with phenytoin (Stores, 1975). Psychotic reactions are described with phenytoin (Glaser, 1972), primidone (Booker, 1972), ethosuximide (Roger et al., 1968), and carbamazepine (Dalby, 1971). In the case of phenytoin, the high blood levels associated with these states are emphasised by Kutt et al. (1964), although idiosyncratic responses often occur shortly after administration of a single dose (Stores, 1975). The psychosis associated with ethosuximide has been recorded in more detail and is of interest. Lorentz de Haas and Stoel (1960) reported three patients who became psychotic on ethosuximide, and in each case during the psychosis, they were free from "absence" seizures. Three other cases reported by Fischer et al. (1965) all had prior psychiatric histories but no clear episodes of psychosis before use of the drug. In these, the relationship of the psychosis to the seizure activity was less clear. Roger et al. (1968) described 15 cases of their own and reviewed other cases in the literature. In 20 cases, paroxysmal EEG changes disappeared; and in 14 cases, normalization of the EEG was seen during the psychotic episodes. It is interesting to note that the average age of the patients was over 22, which is high for patients with petit mal epilepsy, and half of them had had a prior history of psychiatric disorder.

Psychotic behavior precipitated by carbamazepine is interesting in view of the many reports of its beneficial effects on behavior (described below). Thus, Dalby (1971) reported on 5 cases in a series of 51 patients treated with the drug who were withdrawn from the drug due to a worsening of the clinical state. One patient developed schizophreniform illness, which disappeared when the drug was discontinued, and another developed hallucinatory experiences and anxiety attacks as part of the epileptic seizure. Three other patients developed explosiveness with "fits of rage and confusion." All five of these patients had dementia with evidence of cerebral atrophy on pneumo-encephalography.

It is widely known and taught by pediatricians that phenobarbitone may precipitate or aggravate behavior disorders or hyperkinetic syndromes in children (e.g., Ounsted, 1955), but curiously there is no objective study of this phenomenon. Irritability is reported as a side effect of sulthiame (Jeavons, 1975), and sodium valproate is reported to increase hyperactivity in children who are already hyperactive (Barnes and Bower, 1975).

## 1.  Psychoactive Properties

Psychotropic properties have been claimed for several of the anticonvulsants. Phenytoin has been used in the management of both neurotic disorders (Uhlenhuth et al., 1972) and psychosis (Klein and Greenberg, 1967; Simopoulos et al., 1974) with varying effect. However, a direct psychotropic effect is not now recognized. Similar unsubstantiated claims are made for beclamide (Stores, 1975). Primidone is suggested as being useful in the management of hyperactive disorders (Millichap and Fowler, 1967). It is also reported to bring about an "improvement of attitude to environment" and to reduce the incidence of some behavior disorders, in particular neurotic disorders (Von Last, 1972; Trimble et al., 1978a). Phenobarbitone is also related to less neurotic behavior than some other anticonvulsants (Trimble et al., 1978a). Effects of sulthiame on behavior have been more substantially observed and include beneficial effects in personality disorders, improved concentration, motivation, and mood. Reduction in irritability and aggression, decreased viscosity, and improved mental states are also reported (Liu, 1966; Grant, 1974).

Unfortunately, these reports are uncontrolled and subjective. In a longitudinal study of a hyperkinetic girl, Hutt et al. (1966) showed that sulthiame improved behavior, in particular destructive activity. In a study of behavior disorder using rating scales in epileptic children, it was found to be the anticonvulsant drug least associated with conduct disorder (Trimble et al., 1978a). A double-blind controlled study by Moffatt et al. (1970) on 42 subnormal patients randomly allocated to sulthiame and placebo in a crossover design did show that the drug reduced distrubed behavior. Similarly, in a controlled group comparison of 14 subnormal epileptic children and 17 subnormal non-epileptic children, using behavioral rating scales to assess behavior, Al-kaisi and McGuire (1974) demonstrated sulthiame decreased aggressiveness, hyperactivity, destructiveness, and antisocial behavior. This was not dependent on whether the children were epileptic. In the experiments of Dodrill (1975b), an attempt was made to compare phenytoin with sulthiame on a number of indices including social functioning. In this study there were few differences, but those that were significant were in favor of phenytoin, although specific rating scales for mood were not given. A possible reason for lack of confirmation of the other studies was the choice of patients. The controlled trials of sulthiame by Moffatt et al. (1970) and Al-kaisi and McGuire (1974) were carried out on subnormal children.

The drug whose possible psychotropic effects have been described the most is carbamazepine. The literature has recently been reviewed by Dalby (1975): 90 percent of the published reports on the drug mention the psychotropic properties, and collectively 40 reports on 2,000 patients indicate an improvement in seizures in 60 percent and a psychotropic effect in 50 percent. Dalby states:

The psychotropic action is uniformly described as an increase in psychic tempo in patients with the so-called epileptic personality. The slowness, sluggishness, and stickiness, the perseverations and the stereotypies, the apathy and lack of initiative of the patient with long-standing severe epilepsy, usually uncontrolled on large doses of phenobarbital, phenytoin and primidone, diminishes, and a quickening of thought and action occurs. The affective changes, such as irritability, aggressive tendencies, impulsivity, dysphoric episodes, and states of depression and anxiety are reduced or abolished, giving way to an elevation of mood.

Unfortunately, the majority of reports were uncontrolled observations and the studies were primarily concerned with the assessment of seizures. The question has persistently arisen as to whether these effects were due to a psychotropic action of the drug, or to a reduction of other anticonvulsants. Uncontrolled experiments seem to support the idea that it has an independent psychotropic effect in the management of epileptic patients (Daneel, 1967), in behavior disorders in non-epileptic patients (Jacobides, 1966), and in children without epilepsy but with paroxysmal EEG abnormalities and behavior disturbance (Pereira, 1969). But such an effect is not reported in patients on the drug for trigeminal neuralgia (Reynolds, 1975b).

Double-blind trials are much fewer in number, but have been attempted and yield conflicting results. Groh et al. (1971) tested 20 children with carbamazepine and placebo in a crossover design, using 6-week treatment periods separated by therapy-free intervals of 4 weeks. Behavior was rated by questionnaires given to parents and teachers. Carbamazepine was significantly better than placebo at the 5 percent level. De Weis et al. (1974) treated 33 children for 12 weeks on either carbamazepine or placebo. Seventeen received the drug. Fifteen were rated as having excellent or good improvement compared to eight on placebo, a result which was again statistically significant. Unfortunately, the behavior was not objectively rated and few details were given as to which aspects of behavior actually improved. Puente (1975) carried out a double-blind trial on 27 children, comparing carbamazepine to placebo. A variety of behavioral symptoms were rated on a scale of 0 to 4, and those patients whose behavior improved 41 percent or more, were classified as improved. Seventeen improved on carbamazepine and five on placebo. Again, no details were given.

There are five controlled trials in epileptic patients. Rajotte et al. (1967) noted a significant improvement in behavior with carbamazepine as measured on behavior rating scales in a double-blind crossover trial comparing it to placebo. Marjerrison et al. (1968) assessed their patients in a similar way in a trial comparing carbamazepine with phenobarbitone. They reported that patients were less retarded and less often "unhappy" on carbamazepine. In a study of 45 institutionalized patients Cereghino et al. (1974) measured behavior on a rating scale of 53 items completed by ward attendants. They changed patients from their regular medications to carbamazepine, phenobarbitone, or phenytoin. The behavior of more patients deteriorated on phenytoin than on the other drugs, and improvement was seen more in the carbamazepine group. The best changes in behavior were recorded with the phenobarbitone group. Some patients, however, deteriorated in all three drug groups.

In contrast to these results, however, are the negative reports of effects on behavior of Bird et al. (1966) on institutionalized mentally retarded epileptics and Pryse-Phillips and Jeavons (1970) on long-stay mental hospital patients. The former study did not use measurement techniques to assess behavior but relied on assessment by ward staff; however, Pryse-Phillips and Jeavons used rating scales. Twenty-two patients were given either carbamazepine or placebo; and with the drug, a trend was only noted toward a reduction of aggressive behavior and increased ward cooperation. The authors felt that this negative result may have been due to a lower dose of carbamazepine used (600 mg daily) than that used in some other studies. They did not specifically assess changes of mood and so were not assessing a psychotropic effect.

Only one study to date has attempted to assess the relationship of behavior changes to serum carbamazepine levels. In a study of behavior abnormalities in epileptic children it was shown that scores of antisocial behavior obtained from standardized rating scales were negatively correlated with the serum level suggesting a positive psychotropic effect. This was significantly different from the adverse effect phenobarbitone appeared to have on conduct disorder (Trimble et al, 1978a).

In the majority of the above reports on trials in epileptic patients, changes in mood occurred in the absence of any alteration in seizure frequency, and thus the psychotropic effect would seem to be independent from the anticonvulsant effect. The reports of this effect in non-epileptic patients are consistent with this.

## 2.  Comment

It is clear that knowledge of the effects of anticonvulsant drugs on behavior is sparse, and few trials using any form of objective assessment have been conducted. The main ones are summarized in Table 2. If the anecdotal observations are excluded, there is little evidence that anticonvulsant drugs actually make behavior worse and some evidence that sulthiame and carbamazepine have beneficial effects on behavior, in particular aggressive and antisocial behavior. Some drugs may have a beneficial effect on some types of behavior and a deleterious effect on others, such as the differential effect of phenobarbitone in apparently inducing antisocial disorders but perhaps alleviating neurotic disorders. It is clear that much more work needs to be done in this field, in particular using methods of separating out different aspects of behavior and quantifying the results. Studies using serum-anticonvulsant-level estimations are singularly lacking.

## D.  MECHANISM OF INTERFERENCE WITH COGNITIVE FUNCTION AND BEHAVIOR

Clearly, some of the anecdotal reports on the deleterious effects of anticonvulsant drugs refer to acute organic brain syndromes, which present with disorganization of the mental state. However, different mechanisms are presumably responsible for the other effects, in particular for the insidious development of cognitive disabilities. A suggested mechanism in the production of mental changes in epileptic patients is related to the abnormalities of folic-acid metabolism, which have been reported in patients on anticonvulsant drugs. Thus, an association between megaloblastic anemia and anticonvulsant drugs has been recorded, particularly in association with phenytoin (Mannheimer et al., 1952). Additionally, it is recorded with phenobarbitone (Hawkins and Meynell, 1958) and primidone (Chanarin et al., 1958). This is related to folic-acid deficiency, which occurs with these drugs, and for which the etiology is as yet unknown (Reynolds, 1975a). Various theories have been put forward to explain it, including the competitive interaction between folate co-enzymes and the anticonvulsant drugs, malabsorption of folic acid, induction of enzymes involved in folate metabolism, and an increased demand for folic acid as a co-enzyme for anti-epileptic drug hydroxylation (Reynolds, 1975a).

The suggestion that the abnormalities of the mental state seen in epilepsy are related to folate deficiency is supported by observations of an inverse relationship between phenytoin or phenobarbitone serum levels and folate levels in the cerebrospinal (CSF) fluid, an effect greater with phenytoin (Reynolds, 1976). Since the CSF levels of folate are normally three or four times higher than serum levels, it has been suggested that folic acid must

## Table 2. Main Studies of Effects of Anticonvulsant Drugs on Behavior

| Author | Date | No. | Subjects | Control | Duration | Drugs | Serum Levels | Effect on Behavior |
|---|---|---|---|---|---|---|---|---|
| Bird et al. | 1966 | 45 | Retarded epileptics | Yes | 18 mo | Carbamazepine | No | No changes |
| Hutt et al. | 1966 | 1 | Hyperactive | No | — | Sulthiame | No | Improvement |
| Marjerrison et al. | 1968 | 21 | Epileptics | No | 2 mo | Carbamazepine Phenobarbitone | No | Carbamazepine better than phenobarbitone |
| Moffatt et al. | 1970 | 42 | Subnormal | Yes | 6 wk | Sulthiame | No | Reduced disturbed behavior |
| Pryse-Phillips and Jeavons | 1970 | 22 | Epileptics | Yes | 15 wk | Carbamazepine | No | Reduced aggressive behavior with carbamazepine |
| Groh et al. | 1971 | 20 | Children | Yes | 6 wk | Carbamazepine | No | Carbamazepine better than placebo |
| Al-Kaisi and McGuire | 1974 | 18 | Subnormal, epileptic, and non-epileptic | Yes | 3 mo | Sulthiame | No | Decreased aggression and other abnormal behavior |

**Table 2. Main Studies of Effects of Anticonvulsant Drugs on Behavior**

| Author | Date | No. | Subjects | Control | Duration | Drugs | Serum Levels | Effect on Behavior |
|---|---|---|---|---|---|---|---|---|
| Cereghino et al. | 1974 | 45 | Epileptics | No | 3 wk | Carbamazepine Phenobarbitone Phenytoin | No | Phenobarbitone and carbamazepine better than phenytoin |
| de Weis et al. | 1974 | 33 | Children | Yes | 12 wk | Carbamazepine | No | Carbamazepine better than placebo |
| Dodrill | 1975 | 22 | Epileptic adults | No | 6 mo | Phenytoin Sulthiame | No | Phenytoin better than sulthiame on some indices |
| Puente | 1975 | 27 | Children | Yes | 4 wk | Carbamazepine | No | Carbamazepine better than placebo |
| Trimble et al. | 1978a | 312 | Epileptics | No | — | Phenytoin Phenobarbitone Primidone Carbamazepine | Yes | Phenobarbitone and primidone less associated with neurotic disorder. Carbamazepine less associated with conduct disorder. |

have some functional importance in the nervous system (Reynolds, 1976). Disordered metabolism could then be related to the occurrence of the mental symptoms. Further support for this suggestion are observations that psychiatric disturbances, including dementia (Melamed et al., 1975) and schizophreniform psychosis (Reynolds, 1967), as a consequence of folate deficiency have been recognized in non-epileptic patients, and that clinically these conditions have responded to folic-acid therapy. With regard to epileptic patients, it has further been shown that patients with abnormal mental states are more likely to have low-serum folic-acid levels (Reynolds, 1975a), the lowest levels occurring in psychotic and demented patients (Reynolds, 1976). Since some anticonvulsant drugs seem to be more associated with the production of abnormalities in the mental state than others, it is germane to note they the drug most implicated in causing folic-acid distrubances seems to be phenytoin, and that to date carbamazepine has not been implicated in this process. Again the situation with regard to other anticonvulsants has not been properly assessed.

Another mechanism that may explain the production of abnormalities by anticonvulsant drugs is related to their effect on monoamine metabolism. It has been shown experimentally that anticonvulsant drugs increase brain serotonin (Bonneycastle, 1957). Epileptic patients with therapeutic levels of phenytoin, primidone, and phenobarbitone have been reported to have higher CFS levels of the monoamine breakdown products, 5-hydroxy-indole acetic acid (5HIAA) and homovanillic acid (HVA). In addition, patients who are clinically intoxicated have higher levels than those not intoxicated (Chadwick et al., 1975). Since alteration of the mental state can be induced by administration of tryptophan and a monoamine oxidase inhibitor (Oates and Sjoerdsma, 1960), or the serotonin precursor 5-hydroxytryptophan (Trimble et al., 1975), it is possible that such alterations of monoamine metabolism are responsible for the changes in mental state and behavior recorded following the administration of anticonvulsant drugs.

## E.  REFERENCES

Al-Kaisi, A.M., and McGuire, R.J. (1974). The effect of sulthiame on disturbed behaviour in mentally subnormal patients. *Brit. J. Psychiat.* 124:45–49.

Ambrosetto, G., Tassinari, C.A., Baruzzi, A., and Laugaresi, E. (1977). Phenytoin encephalopathy as a probable idiosyncratic reaction. *Epilepsia.* 18:405–408.

Barnes, M. ., and Fetterman, J.N. (1938). Mentality of dispensary epileptic patients. *Arch. Neurol. Psychiat.* 40:903–910.

Barnes, S.E., and Bower, B.D. (1975). Sodium valproate in the treatment of intractable childhood epilepsy. *Devel. Med. Child Neurol.* 17:175–181.

Bird, C.A.K., Griffin, B.P., Miklascewska, J.M., and Galbraith, A.W. (1966). Tegretol: A controlled trial of a new anticonvulsant. *Brit. J. Psychiat.* 112:737–742.

Bonduelle, M., Bouygues, P., Sallou, C., and Chemal, Y.R. (1964). Clinical trials of an antiepileptic drug G32883. Results of 89 observations. III. Congress of International College of Neuropharmacology. Munich 1962. Elsevier, Amsterdam. pp. 312–316.

Bonneycastle, D.D., Giarman, N.J., and Paasonen, M.K. (1957). Anticonvulsant compounds and 5-hydroxytryptamine in rat brain. *Brit. J. Pharmacol.* 12:228–231.

Booker, H.E. (1972). Primidone: Toxicity, in *Antiepileptic Drugs*. D.M. Woodbury, J.K. Penry, and R.P. Schmidt, eds. Raven Press, New York.

Booker, H.E., Matthews, C.G., and Slaby, A. (1967). Effects of diphenylhydantoin on selected physiological-psychological measures in normal adults. *Neurol.* 17:949–951.

Boxer, C.M., Herzberg, J.L., and Scott, D.F. (1976). Has sodium valproate hypnotic effects? *Epilepsia.* 17:367–370.

Browne, T.R., Dreifuss, F.E., Dyken, P.R., Goode, D.J., Penry, J.K. Porter, R.J., White, B.J., and White, P.T. (1975). Ethosuximide in the treatment of absence (petit mal) seizures. *Neurol.* 25:515–525.

Cereghino, J.J., Brock, J.T., Van Meter, J.C., Penry, J.R., Smith, L.D., and White, B.G. (1974). Carbamazepine for epilepsy. *Neurol.* 24:401–410.

Chadwick, D., Jenner, P., and Reynolds, E.H. (1975). Amines, anticonvulsants, and epilepsy. *Lancet.* 1:473–476.

Chanarin, I., Elvas, P.C., and Mollin, D.L. (1958). Folic acid studies in megaloblastic anaemia due to primidone. *Brit. Med. J.* 2:80–82.

Chaudhry, M.R., and Pond, D.A. (1961). Mental deterioration in epileptic children. *J. Neurol. Neurosurg. Psychiat.* 24:213–219.

Dalby, M.A. (1975). Behavioural effects of carbamazepine, in *Advances in Neurology II.* J.K. Penry and D.D. Daly, eds. Raven Press, New York.

Dalby, M.A. (1971). Antiepileptic and psychotropic effect of carbamazepine in the treatment of psychomotor epilepsy. *Epilepsia.* 12:325–334.

Daneel, A.B. (1967). Tegretol in institutionalised epileptics. *S. Afr. Med. J.* 41:772–775.

de Weis, M.L.M., de Monk, C.G., Chardon, M.C., and Waitz, A.M. (1974). Entoque diagnostico y terapeutico del "nino turbulento." *Sem. Med.* 144:9.

Dodrill, C.B. (1975a). DPH serum levels, toxicity, and neuropsychological performance in patients with epilepsy. *Epilepsia.* 16:593–600.

Dodrill, C.B. (1975b). Effects of sulthiame upon intellectual, neuropsychological, and social functioning abilities among adult epileptics: Comparison with diphenylhydantoin. *Epilepsia.* 16:617–625.

Finkleman, I., and Arieff, A.J. (1942). Untoward effects of phenytoin sodium in epilepsy. *J.A.M.A.* 118:1209–1212.

Fischer, M., Korskjaer, G., and Pedersen, E. (1965). Psychotic episodes in Zarondan treatment. *Epilepsia.* 6:325–334.

Fox, J.T. (1924). Response of epileptic children to mental and educational tests. *Brit. J. Med. Psychol.* 4:235–248.

Frantzen, E., Hansen, J.M., Hansen, O.E., Kristensen, M. (1967). Phenytoin intoxication. *Acta Neurolog. Scand.* 43:440–446.

Glaser, G.H. (1972). Diphenylhydantoin toxicity, in *Antiepileptic Drugs*. D.M. Woodbury, J.K. Penry, and R.P. Schmidt, eds. Raven Press, New York.

Goode, D.J., Penry, J.K., and Dreifuss, F.E. (1970). Effect of paroxysmal spike wave on continuous visual motor performance. *Epilepsia.* 11:241–254.

Gowers, W.R. (1885). *Epilepsy and Other Chronic Convulsive Diseases: Their Causes, Symptoms, and Treatment.* William Wood, London.

Grant, R.H.E. (1974). Sulthiame and behaviour. *Devel. Med. Child Neurol.* 16:821–824.

Green, J.R., Troupon, A.S., Halpern, L.M., Friel, P., and Kanarek, P. (1974). Sulthiame: Evaluation as an anticonvulsant. *Epilepsia.* 15:329–349.

Grinker, R.R. (1929). The proper use of phenobarbital in the treatment of the epilepsies. *J.A.M.A.* 93:1218-1219.

Groh, C.L., Rosenmayr, F., and Birnbaumer, N. (1971). Psychotrope Wirkung von Carbamazepine bie nicht epileptischen. *Kind. Med. Monats.* 25:329-333.

Guerrant, J., Anderson, W.W., Fischer, A., Weinstein, M.R., Jarros, R.M., and Deskins, A. (1962). *Personality in Epilepsy.* Charles C. Thomas, Springfield.

Guey, J., Charles, C., Coquery, C., Roger, J., and Soulayrol, R. (1967). Study of psychological effect of ethosoximide on 25 children suffering from petit mal epilepsy. *Epilepsia.* 8:129-141.

Haerer, A.F., and Grace, J.B. (1969). Studies of anticonvulsant levels in epileptics. *Acta Neurolog. Scand.* 45:18-31.

Hawkins, C.F., and Meynell, M.J. (1958). Macrocytosis and macrocytic anaemia caused by anticonvulsant drugs. *Quart. J. Med.* 27:45-63.

Holdsworth, L., and Whitmore, K. (1974). A study of children with epilepsy attending ordinary schools. *Devel. Med. Child Neurol.* 16:746-758.

Husby, J. (1963). Delayed toxicity and serum concentrations of phenytoin. *Dan. Med. Bull.* 10:236-239.

Hutt, C., Jackson, P.M., and Level, M. (1966). Behavioural parameters and drug effects. *Epilepsia.* 7:250-259.

Hutt, S.J., Jackson, P.M., Belsham, A., and Higgins, G. (1968). Perceptual motor behaviour in relation to blood phenobarbitone level. A preliminary report. *Devel. Med. Child Neurol.* 10:626-632.

Ideström, C.M., Schalling, D., Calquist, U., and Sjoquist, F. (1972). Acute effects of diphenylhydantoin in relation to plasma levels. Behavioural and psychological studies. *Psycholog. Med.* 2:111-120.

Jacobides, G.M. (1966). New uses and some abuses of carbamyldibenzazepine (Tegretol) as a psychotropic agent. Proceedings of the IV World Cbngress of Psychiatry, Madrid.

Jeavons, P.M. (1975). The practical management of epilepsy. *Hosp. Update.* 1:11-18.

Kerfriden, P. (1970). Effets psychiques defavorable des medications anticonvitiales. *Rev. Neuropsychiat. Infantile.* 18:605-609.

Klein, O.F., and Greenberg, I.M. (1967). Behavioural effects of DPH in severe psychiatric disorders. *Am. J. Psychiat.* 124:847 849.

Kooiker, J.C., and Sumi, S.M. (1974). Movement disorder as a manifestation of DPH intoxication. *Neurol.* 24:68-71.

Krasovsky, J., Villanueva, R., and Hernandez, O. (1972). La carbamazepine en el tratemiento sintomatico de los trastornos de conducta infantil. *Munch. Med. Wochen.* 114:619-622.

Kutt, H., Winters, W., Kokenge, R., and McDowell, F. (1964). Diphenylhydantoin metabolism, blood levels and toxicity. *Arch. Neurol.* 11:642-648.

Lennox, W.G. (1942). Brain injury, drugs, and environment as a cause of mental decay in epilepsy. *Am. J. Psychiat.* 99:174-180.

Lennox, W.G., and Lennox, M.A. (1960). *Epilepsy and Related Disorders.* Little, Brown & Co., Boston.

Liu, M.C. (1966). Clinical experience with sulthiame. *Brit. J. Psychiat.* 112:621-628.

Livingston, S. (1972). *Drug Therapy for Epilepsy.* Charles C. Thomas, Springfield.

Logan, W.J., and Freeman, J.M. (1969). Pseudodegenerative disease due to diphenylhydantoin intoxication. *Arch. Neurol.* 21:631-637.

Lorentz de Haas, A.M., and Stoel, L.M.K. (1960). Experiences with α ethyl α methylsuccinimide in the treatment of epilepsy. *Epilepsia.* 1:501-511.

Loveland, N., Smith, B., and Forster, F. (1957). Mental and emotional changes in epileptic patients on continuous anticonvulsant medication. *Neurol.* 7:856-865.

Mannheimer, E., Packesch, F., Reimer, E.E., and Vetter, H. (1952). Die Haematolgischen

Komplikationen der Epilepsiebehandlung mit Hydantoin-korpem. *Med. Klinik.* 47:1397–1401.

Marjerrison, G., Jedlicki, S.M., Keogh, R.P., Hrychuk, W., and Poulakakis, G.M. (1968). Carbamazepine: Behavioural, anticonvulsant, and EEG effects in chronically hospitalised epileptics. *Dis. Ner. Syst.* 29:133–136.

Matthews, C.G., and Harley, J.P. (1975). Differential psychological test performances in toxic and nontoxic adult epileptics. *Neurol.* 25:184–188.

McLellan, D.L., and Swash, M. (1974). Choreoathetosis and encephalopathy induced by phenytoin. *Brit. Med. J.* 2:204–205.

Melamed, E., Reches, A., and Hershko, C. (1975). Reversible cerebral nervous system dysfunction in folate deficiency. *J. Neurolog. Sci.* 25:93–98.

Merritt, H.H. (1955). *A Textbook of Neurology.* Lea and Febiger, Philadelphia.

Millichap, J.G., and Fowler, G.W. (1967). Treatment of "minimal brain dysfunction" syndromes. *Paed. Clin. N. Am.* 14:767–777.

Moffatt, W.R., Siddiqui, A.R., and Mackay, D.N. (1970). The use of sulthiame with disturbed mentally subnormal patients. *Brit. J. Psychiat.* 117:673–678.

Niedermeyer, E., Blumer, D., Holscher, E., and Walker, B.A. (1970). Classical hysterical seizures precipitated by anticonvulsant toxicity. *Psychiatrica Clinica.* 3:71.

Oates, J.A., and Sjoerdsma, A. (1960). Neurological effects of tryptophan in patients receiving a monoamine oxidase inhibitor. *Neurol.* 10:1076–1078.

Ounstead, C. (1955). The hyperkinetic syndrome in epileptic children. *Lancet.* 2:303–311.

Parsonage, M. (1975). Treatment with carbamazepine: Adults, in *Advances in Neurology, Vol 11.* J.K. Penry and D.D. Daly, eds. Raven Press, New York.

Patel, H., and Crichton, J.V. (1968). The neurologic hazards of diphenylhydantoin in childhood. *J. Paed.* 73:676–684.

Pereira, J.L.C. (1969). Nossa experiencia com o tegretol nas manifestaçones comiciais não convulsivas da infância. *O. Hosp.* 75:687–692.

Perlo, V.P., and Schwab, R.S. (1969). Unrecognized dilantin intoxication, in *Modern Neurology,* S Locke, ed. Little, Brown & Co., Boston. pp. 589–597.

Prensky, A.L., De Vivo, D.C., and Palkes, H. (1971). Severe bradykinesia as a manifestation of toxicity to antiepileptic medication. *J. Paed.* 78:700–704.

Pryse-Phillips, W.E.M., and Jeavons, P.M. (1970). Effect of carbamazepine on the electroencephalographic and ward behaviour of patients with chronic epilepsy. *Epilepsia.* 11:263–273.

Puente, R.M. (1975). The use of carbamazepine in the treatment of behavioural disorders in children, In *Epileptic Seizures—Behaviour—Pain* W. Birkmayer, ed. Hans Huber, Stuttgart.

Rajotte, P., Jilek, L., Perales, A., Giard, N., Bordeleau, J.M., and Tetreault, L. (1967). Proprietés antiepileptiques et psychotropes de la carbamazepine. *Union Med. Canada.* 96:1200–1206.

Rawson, M.D. (1968). Diphenylhydantoin intoxication and cerebrospinal fluid protein. *Neurol.* 18:1009–1011.

Rett, A. (1976). The so-called psychotropic effect of tegretol in the treatment of convulsions of cerebral origin in children, In *Epileptic Seizures—Behaviour—Pain.* W. Birkmayer, ed. Hans Huber, Stuttgart.

Reynolds, E.H. (1967). Schizophrenia-like psychoses of epilepsy and disturbances of folate and B12 metabolism induced by anticonvulsant drugs. *Brit. J. Psychiat.* 113:911–919.

Reynolds, E.H. (1970). Iatrogenic disorders in epilepsy, in *Modern Trends in Neurology No. 5.* D. Williams, ed. Butterworth, London. pp. 271–286.

Reynolds, E.H. (1975a). Chronic antiepileptic toxicity: A review. *Epilepsia.* 16:319–353.

Reynolds, E.H. (1975b). In discussion: Behavioural effects of carbamazepine, in *Advances in Neurology Vol 11.* J.K. Penry and D.D. Daly, eds. Raven press, New York. p. 343.

Reynolds, E.H. (1976). Neurological aspects of folate and B12 metabolism. *Clin. Haematol.* 5:661-694.

Reynolds, E.H., and Travers, R. (1974). Serum anticonvulsant concentrations in epileptic patients with mental symptoms. *Brit. J. Psychiat.* 124:440-445.

Rodin, E.A., Rim, C.S., Kitano, H., Lewis, R., and Rennick, P.M. (1976). A comparison of the effectiveness of primidone versus carbamazepine in epileptic outpatients. *J. Nerv. Ment. Dis.* 163:41-46.

Roger, J., Grangeon, H., Guey, J., and Lob, H. (1968). Psychiatric and psychological effects of ethosuximide treatment in epileptics. *Encephale.* 57:407-438.

Roseman, E. (1961). Dilantin toxicity. *Neurol.* 11:912-921.

Rosen, J.A. (1968). Dilantin dementia. *Trans. Am. Neurolog. Assn.* 93:273.

Royo, D., and Martin, F. (1959). Standardized psychometrical tests applied to the analysis of the effects of anticonvulsant medication on the intellectual proficiency of young epileptics. *Epilepsia.* 1:189-207.

Schain, R.J., Ward, J.W., and Guthrie, D. (1977). Carbamazepine as an anticonvulsant in children. *Neurol.* 27:476-480.

Schlack, H.G. (1974). Ergenyl in the treatment of epilepsy. *Therapiewoche.* 24:39.

Simopoulos, A.M., Pinto, A., Uhlenhuth, E.H., McGee, J.J., and de Rosa, E.R. (1974). D.P.H. effectiveness in the treatment of chronic schizophrenics. *Arch. Gen. Psychiat.* 30:106-111.

Smith, W.L., Philipus, M.J., and Guard, H.L. (1968). Psychometric study of children with learning problems and 14 positive spike EEG patterns, treated with ethosuximide (zarontin) and placebo. *Arch. Dis. Childhood.* 43:616-619.

Smyth, V.O.G. (1964). The use of ospolot in temporal lobe epilepsy. *Epilepsia.* 5:293-295.

Somerfeld-Ziskind, E., and Ziskind, E. (1940). Effect of phenobarbital on the mentality of epileptic patients. *Arch. Neurol. Psychiat.* 43:70-79.

Soulayrol, R., and Rbger, J. (1970). Effets psychiatriques defavourables des medicacions antiepileptiques. *Rev. Neuropsychiat. Infantile.* 18:599-603.

Stores, G. (1975). Behavioural effects of anticonvulsant drugs. *Devel. Med. Child Neurol.* 17:647-658.

Tchicaloff, M., and Gaillard, F. (1970). Quelques effets indesirables des medicaments antiepileptiques sur les rendements intellectuels. *Rev. Neuropsychiat. Infantile.* 18:599-603.

Tempkin, O. (1971). *The Falling Sickness.* Johns Hopkins, Baltimore.

Trimble, M.R. and Corbett, J. (1978a): The effects of anticonvulsant drugs on behaviour. (In preparation.)

Trimble, M.R. and Corbett, J. (1978b). The effects of anticonvulsant drugs on cognitive function. (In preparation.)

Trimble, M.R., Chadwick, D., Reynolds, E.H., and Marsden, C.D. (1975). L-5-hydroxytryptophan and mood. *Lancet.* 1:583.

Uhlenhuth, E.H., Stephens, J.H., Dim, B.H., and Covi, L. (1972). D.P.H. and phenobarbital in the relief of psychoneurotic symptoms. *Psychopharmacologia.* 27:67.

Vallarta, J.M., Bell, D.B., and Reichert, A. (1974). Progressive encephalopathy due to chronic hydantoin intoxication. *Am. J. Dis. Childhood.* 128:27-34.

Von Last, G. (1972). Epilepsie—Behandlung mit Mylepsinum. *Allemeinmedizin/der Landarzt.* 7:336-341.

Wapner, I., Thurston, D.L., and Holowach, J. (1962). Phenobarbital: Its effects on learning in epileptic children. *J.A.M.A.* 182:937.

Weiss, C.F., Heffelfinger, J.C., and Buchanan, R.A. (1969). Serial dilantin levels in mentally retarded children. *Am. J. Ment. Def.* 73:826-830.

Woodbury, D.M., Penry, J.K., and Schmidt, R.P., eds. 1972. *Antiepileptic Drugs.* Raven Press, New York.

Current Developments in Psychopharmacology, Volume 6
© 1981, Spectrum Publications, Inc.

# CHAPTER 4

# DRUG-INDUCED TARDIVE DYSKINESIA

## HITOSHI ITOH

Drug-induced tardive dyskinesia, which occurs in the course of long-term administration of psychotropic drugs, especially neuroleptics, and persists for years even after drug removal, began to be reported in the late 1950s. Since then, more than 100 investigations on this subject have been described. And it is estimated that 10 to 30 percent of long-term hospitalized psychiatric patients in Europe and North America exhibit tardive dyskinesia, whereas 5 to 20 percent of patients exhibit this syndrome in Japan. These findings suggest that the manifestation of tardive dyskinesia will become a serious problem in the investigation of psychotropic drug treatment.

The author presents a review of the symptomatology, etiological factors, differential diagnosis, prognosis, and management of this syndrome. Results of the author's studies in the cross-national survey and on the reversibility of tardive dyskinesia are also described.

In connection with biochemical theory of the etiology of tardive dyskinesia, a variety of therapeutic investigations have been carried out, but no successful therapy could be found among them. Therefore, the author stresses that the early diagnosis of dyskinetic symptoms, possible removal of responsible drugs, and preventive care in daily psychotropic drug treatment are regarded as extremely important in the management of this syndrome.

## A. INTRODUCTION

The new type of involuntary movements observed in patients under long-term administration of neuroleptics has come into notice in Europe and North America since the late 1950s and is now generally referred to as "tardive dyskinesia." In 1952—the year after the introduction of chlorpromazine to the treatment—it was noted that transient extrapyramidal symptoms, such as Parkinsonism, akathisia, and acute dystonic reaction appeared in the earlier stages of neuroleptic treatment. However, tardive dyskinesia occurs a few months or years after the antipsychotic drug treatment and is characterized by: (1) peculiar dyskinetic involuntary movements of the perioral region, occasionally expanding to the neck, extremities, and trunk; (2) a tendency to persist and often to become permanent or irreversible, even after the discontinuation of causal neuroleptic medication; and (3) poor response to anti-Parkinsonian agents. In some cases, the dyskinetic movements do not disappear despite drug withdrawal; or they first appear with reduction or discontinuation of neuroleptics. After recognition of tardive dyskinesia, the classification of "drug-induced extrapyramidal symptoms" was revised as follows:

1. Drug-induced Parkinsonism or pseudo-parkinsonism*
2. Akathisia
3. Acute dystonic reactions
   a. Dystonia
   b. Dyskinesia
4. Tardive dyskinesia**

The persistence of an extrapyramidal symptom such as Parkinsonism or dystonia after removal of psychotropic drugs was reported by Schönecker (1956) and Ey and Rappard (1956). Sigwald et al. (1959) believed that these persistent involuntary movements caused by psychotropic drugs should be separated as an independent syndrome and referred to as "dyskinesia facio-linguo-masticatrice." Uhrbrand and Faurbye (1960) also reported that persistent involuntary movements of the face and/or extremities occurred after long-term treatments with perphenazine, chlorpromazine, reserpine, and also electro-shock; and they named these movements "irreversible dyskinesia."

Subsequently, many different terms explaining this syndrome were devised; for example, "das terminale extrapyramidale Insuffizienz- bzw. Defekt-Syndrom" (Haddenbrock, 1965), "persistierende extrapyramidale Hyperkinesen" (Degwitz et al., 1967), persistent oral dyskinesia (Hunter et al., 1968), tardive dyskinesia (Faurbye et al., 1964; Crane, 1968), and "späte

---

* including Akinesia.
** including rabbit syndrome.

extrapyramidale Hyperkinesen" (Hippius and Lange, 1970). But today the term "tardive dyskinesia" is commonly and is not always a definite neurological word. It is sometimes used for representing general extrapyramidal motor disorders, including akathisia and bradykinesia (Curzon, 1968); but in general, it signifies hyperkinesia as an extrapyramidal symptom or, in particular, hyperkinesia with characteristic abnormality.

From the late 1950s to 1977, more than 100 reports on this subject have been described, and the clinical features, etiology, epidemiology, and management of the syndrome have been reviewed in detail by some investigators (Crane, 1968, 1973, 1975; Kazamatsuri et al., 1971, 1972; Klawans, 1973; Tarsy and Baldessarini, 1976; Parks, 1976; Bourgeois, 1977; Simpson and Kline, 1976; and others). Recently, a variety of therapeutic studies have been carried out on this syndrome, in connection with biochemical theory that the etiology of tardive dyskinesia may be related to the blockade of dopamine and other neurochemical transmitters by neuroleptics.

In Japan, the existence of this syndrome was first noticed in the late 1960s, and the first patient with tardive dyskinesia was reported by Yagi, in November 1970. Results of the subsequent survey studies on tardive dyskinesia in mental hospitals in Japan (Itoh et al., 1971; Kinoshita, 1972; Karasuyama, 1972); those of the cross-national survey study both in France and Japan (Ogita et al. 1972); and results of the comparative survey between Japan and the United States (Kazamatsuri, 1971) demonstrated that the prevalence of this syndrome in Japan was similar (5 to 20 percent) to that in European countries.

In the United States, a special report on the subject was published (ACNP—FDA, 1973). At the same time, all makers of antipsychotic drugs in the United States updated their package inserts to include information on persistent dyskinesia, and cautioned all physicians in the use of neuroleptics (Cole, 1975). Similar action was taken in Japan: The information on tardive dyskinesia was requested to be included in the package inserts of all marketed neuroleptics.

Considering the possibility that tardive dyskinesia may develop from the use of long-term administration of neuroleptics, together with the fact that results of neuroleptic therapy—from the standpoint of the long-term prognosis of chronic psychiatric diseases—have not met our initial expectations, we should review the current status of pharmacotherapy on psychotics and organize urgent preventive measures against tardive dyskinesia caused by neuroleptic treatment.

Since symposiums on tardive dyskinesia have been held at CINP (Collegium Internationale Neuro-Psychopharmacologicum), WPA (World Psychiatric Association), and many other international congresses for several years, the author would like to review the newly reported topics and investigations in Japan.

## B. PREVALENCE OF TARDIVE DYSKINESIA

The prevalence of tardive dyskinesia in hospitalized patients has been reported by many investigators. (See Table 1.) Some reasons for the varying range of occurrences (0.5 to 56 percent) might depend on: (1) the patient's background characteristics, (2) the drug status, (3) the procedure of investigation, or (4) the criteria and accuracy of judgment.

For example, in 1971, when we first conducted a survey study on the occurrence of tardive dyskinesia among 2,940 hospitalized patients in 6 mental hospitals around Tokyo, we found only 10 irreversible and severe cases (0.3 percent). But as a result of a subsequent survey, more patients with tardive dyskinesia were found in these institutions; consequently the prevalence increased to 4 or 5 percent. Nearly 50 cases with severe dyskinetic movements among them were recorded in the movie.

According to an investigation by Yagi et al. in 1972, the prevalence of tardive dyskinesia amounted to 12.5 percent, excluding 7 suspicious cases.

Ogita surveyed the hospitalized patients in Hôpital Psychiatrique de Bassens (France) and found that 22 of the patients under neuroleptic treatment had persistent dyskinesia (prevalence rate 18.3 percent). In 1972, after he returned from France, Ogita observed the presence of persistent dyskinesia in Inogashira Hospital on the basis of the same diagnostic criteria, and it was found that 22 of 123 cases (17.9 percent) exhibited this syndrome (Ogita et al., 1975).

Summarizing the reuslts shown in Table 1, it is estimated that 10 to 30 percent of long-term hospitalized psychiatric patients in Europe and North America exhibit tardive dyskinesia, whereas 5 to 20 percent exhibit this syndrome in Japan. As a result of our study, it seems that there is fundamentally no marked difference in the prevalence of the syndrome among the races.

## C. CLINICAL FEATURES AND LOCALIZATION

The main characteristic of tardive dyskinesia is involuntary movement around the mouth. In the patients receiving long-term neuroleptic administration, vermicular movement of the tongue, tic-like involuntary movement of facial muscles, and abnormal movements of the neck and/or jaw are most frequently observed as early symptoms. Ayd emphasized that prompt withdrawal of responsible neuroleptics at this stage could prevent these dyskinetic movements from progressing to the chronic or irreversible stage, but careful attention is necessary to stop the progression at this particular point.

If the dyskinetic movements are advanced, BLM syndrome (Bucco-Lingo-Masticatory syndrome) becomes notable; it is characterized by

## Table 1. Prevalence of Tardive Dyskinesia

| Author(s) | Year | Prevalence* | Institution(s) | Country |
|---|---|---|---|---|
| Faurbye et al. | 1964 | 26.1% (109/417) | St. Hans Hospital | Denmark |
| Turunen and Achté | 1967 | 5.0% (24/480) | 2 hospitals in Kupittaa | Finland |
| Haddenbrock | 1966 | 3.0% (30/900) | Emmendinger Krankenhaus | West Germany |
| Degwitz et al. | 1966 | 16.9% (130/766) | Goddellau Psychiatrische Psychiatrische | West Germany |
| Degwitz et al. | 1966 | 25.7% (114/443) | Krankenhaus Giessen | West Germany |
| Degwitz et al. | 1966 | 13.8% (43/312) | Psychiatrische Krankenhaus Peppenheim | West Germany |
| Hippius and Lange | 1970 | 30.1% (201/668) | Karl-Bonhoeffer Nervenklinik | West Germany |
| Heinrich et al. | 1968 | 13.0% (98/755) | | West Germany |
| Eckman, F. | 1968 | 3.0% (43/1441) | | West Germany |
| Hoff and Hoffman | 1967 | 0.5% (46/10019) | 14 mental hospitals | Austria, West Germany, and Switzerland |
| Lambert | 1970 | 25.0% | | France |
| Ogita et al. | 1971 | 18.3% (24/131) | Hôpital Psychiatrique de Bassens | France |
| Bourgeois | 1977 | 8.2% (258/3140) | 4 mental hospitals in Aquitaine | France |
| Hunter et al. | 1964 | 2.8% (13/450) | The National Hospital | U.K. |

## Table 1. (Cont'd)

| Author(s) | Year | Prevalence* | Institution(s) | Country |
|---|---|---|---|---|
| Edwards and Pryce | 1966 | 17.0% (21/120) | Whitchurch Hospital | U.K. |
| Demars | 1966 | 7.0% (34/488) | Towers Hospital | U.K. |
| Edwards | 1970 | 27.2% (50/184) | A mental hospital | U.K. |
| Brandon et al. | 1971 | 24.0% (150/625) | St. Nicolas Hospital | U.K. |
| Kennedy et al. | 1971 | 39.7% (25/63) | Naburn and Bootham Hospital | U.K. |
| Sied and Müller | 1967 | 11.4% (46/404) | Douglous Hospital | Canada |
| Villeneuve et al. | 1969 | 2.2% (68/3280) | St. Michael–Archange Hospital | Canada |
| Lehman et al. | 1970 | 6.6% (23/350) | Douglous Hospital | Canada |
| Roxburgh | 1970 | 2.5% (3/120) | University of Albert Hospital | Canada |
| Crane and Paulson | 1967 | 15.0% (27/182) | Dorothea Dix State Hospital | U.S.A. |

| Author | Year | Percentage* | Location | Country |
|---|---|---|---|---|
| Paulson | 1968 | 10.0% (50/500) | | U.S.A. |
| Greenblatt et al. | 1968 | 38.5% (20/52) | | U.S.A. |
| Crane | 1968 | 27.7% (105/379) | 5 state hospitals | U.S.A. |
| Crane and Chase | 1970 | 27.0% (34/127) | Dorothea Dix State Hospital | U.S.A. |
| Dynes | 1970 | 9.0% (103/1200) | V.A. hospital, Salem, Va. | U.S.A. |
| Ettinger and Curran | 1970 | 1.0% (10/1000) | | U.S.A. |
| Kazamatsuri | 1971 | 14.9% (25/170) | Boston State Hospital | U.S.A. |
| Fann et al. | 1972 | 36.0% | V.A. hospitals & state hospital in Tennessee | U.S.A. |
| Itoh et al. | 1971 | 0.3% (10/2940) | 10 mental hospitals in Tokyo | Japan |
| Ogita et al. | 1972 | 17.9% (22/123) | Inogashira Hospital | Japan |
| Yagi | 1972 | 12.5% (7/56) (25.0% (14/56)) | Minagawa Hospital | Japan |
| Sakai et al. | 1972 | 14.1% (56/396) | 3 mental hospitals in Kanagawa | Japan |
| Karasuyama et al. | 1973 | 7.2% (33/463) | 2 mental hospitals in Nagasaki | Japan |

* (Number of administered cases/total number of patients with tardive dyskinesia).

repetitive, stereotyped involuntary movements of the tongue, lips, facial muscles, and jaw—similar to Huntington's chorea—and some cases are accompanied by choreo-athetotic movements of the extremities and axial involuntary movements of the trunk or rotatory pelvic movements. The severe cases sometimes exhibit abnormal movements, such as ballisms or myoclony; or those with hypertonic features, such as torsions dystony or torticollis.

There is a wide variety of involuntary movements in tardive dyskinesia. Facial and oral movements are most frequently observed and may be presented as frowning, blinking, smiling, and grimacing in the forehead, eyebrows, periorbital area or cheeks; as puckering, pouting, smacking of the lips; as biting, clenching, chewing, mouth opening, lateral movements of the jaw; as rhythmical rolling, backward and forward movements, or lateral movements of the tongue.

The abnormal movements often observed in a patient's trunk and extremities are: rocking, twisting, and squirming of the neck, shoulders, hips, and abdomen; pelvic gyrations; anterior posterior body rocking; strange choreic or athetoid movements of the upper extremities; lateral knee movements, foot tapping, heel dropping, foot squirming, or inversion and eversion of the foot.

The peculiar involuntary movements of this syndrome are variously named. For example, the facial and oral movements are referred to as fly-catching syndrome, oral dyskinesia, "orale Unruhe," Bucco-Linguo-Masticatory syndrome (BLM syndrome), and "dyskinesia linguo-bucco-masticatrice." Dyskinesia involving the respiratory muscles leads to disturbance of respiratory rhythm, and is termed respiratory dyskinesia, or "Atemrhythmus-störungen." "Schulter-hochziehen," for the movements of the extremities and trunk, means raising the shoulders and drawing in the neck; rocking movement means shaking the trunk; "manuale Leeraktivität" explains the meaningless movements of the fingers and hands; and "Unruhe in den Beinen" signifies the continuous movements of the lower extremities.

Although tardive dyskinesia consists of persistent involuntary movements, the type and severity of the symptoms are changeable under different conditions. Crane (1975) enumerated the patient's alertness, motion, posture, and drug status as potent influential factors. Dyskinetic movements disappear during sleep and decrease or weaken when the patient's alertness lessens. On the other hand, these movements increase and strengthen under such conditions of heightened alertness, such as agitation, overt anxiety, or increased vigilance. As for motion, the particular behaviors increasing the associated movements enhance tardive dyskinesia. For example, abnormal facial movements, dyskinesia of the hands, or dystonia of the upper extremities are identified more markedly during walking than when in a state of repose; and oro-facial dyskinesia increases during finger-tapping. By making use of this method, it is possible to induce and find very slight or masked dyskinesia. Also, during conversation, dyskinesia of the facial muscles disappears, while that of hands and feet strengthen, and the involuntary movement of hands decreases while the hands are in use. This suggests that dyskinesia tends to be controlled in the exercising parts and enhanced in the remote parts. With regard to posture, dyskinesia appears more remarkably in the standing position than in the sitting or supine position. Concerning the drug status, drug-induced Parkinsonism, akathisia, and acute dystonic reactions are relieved or disappear by reduction in dosage or discontinuation of antipsychotic drugs; but on the other hand, dyskinesia is rather enhanced.

In some cases, tardive dyskinesia does not appear during long-term neuroleptic treatment, but may first appear after dosage reduction or drug withdrawal. This type of dyskinesia is called "withdrawal dyskinesia."

Table 2 shows sites and characteristics of tardive dyskinesia, including the results of investigation by Ogita et al. at Hôpital Psychiatrique de Bassens (France) and at Inogashira Hospital (Japan), as well as those of surveys in Japan by Yagi et al. (1976), Kinoshita (1973), and others. The majority of cases showed oral dyskinesia with abnormal movements of the mouth, cheeks, tongue, and jaw (96.7 percent), with some cases accompanied by involuntary movements of the upper and lower extremities and neck and trunk (34.9 percent). There are very few cases showing dyskinetic movements localized in portions other than the perioral area (3.3 percent).

In the absence of oral dyskinesia, Choreo-athetose-like movements of the extremities were found in 16.6 percent of the cases, body-weight-shifting phenomenon in 7.3 percent, abnormal movements of the neck in 4.6 percent (torticollis, dystonia, repetitive movements), tic-like movements of the face in 2 cases, and tremor of the upper extremities in 1 case.

Villeneuve (1969) classified tardive dyskinesia into 4 types, as follows: (1) syndrome choreiforme, (2) syndrome bucco-linguale, (3) syndrome bucco-facio-linguale, and (4) rabbit syndrome. Kazamatsuri (1972) also divided it into the following 4 types: (1) lingual dyskinesia, (2) linguo-masticatory dyskinesia, (3) bucco-oral dyskinesia, and (4) choreoathetotic dyskinesia. However, clinical cases of tardive dyskinesia observed in daily practice are varied, and frequently, various kinds of dyskinetic movements exist concomitantly; therefore, it is not always possible to classify the syndrome as precisely as described above.

Most patients with tardive dyskinesia neither become aware of dyskinetic movements, nor are they distressed by them. As Crane (1975) described, most patients admitted to mental hospitals are chronic schizophrenic or senile patients, who are in half-asleep conditions most of the time. Therefore, their alertness lessens, and abnormal movements do not tend to occur.

At the same time, since the patients are unconcerned with themselves

Table 2. Patients With Tardive Dyskinesia (Affected Regions)

| Author | No. of Patients | Number of Patients (%) | | | Features of Dyskinetic Movement Other than Oral Dyskinesia |
| | | With Oral Dyskinesia (Dyskinesia Facio-Linguo-Masticatrice) | With Oral Dyskinesia + Dyskinesia of Other Regions | With Dyskinesia Other than Oral Dyskinesia | |
|---|---|---|---|---|---|
| (1) Itoh | 10 | 1 (10%) | 5 (50%) | 4 (40%) | Choreo-athetotic form 7<br>Torticollis 3<br>Myoclony-like movement 1 |
| (2) Ogita (France) | 24 | 16 (66.7%) | 8 (33.3%) | 0 | Balance (constant shifting of weight from one foot to the other) 6<br>Athetose-like movement of the upper extremity 2<br>"Dandinement" (constant rocking of head forward and backward) 2 |

| | | | | | | |
|---|---|---|---|---|---|---|
| (5) Ogita | 22 | 5 (68.2%) | 7 (31.8%) | 0 | Balance | 3 |
| | | | | | Athetose-like movement of the hand | 1 |
| | | | | | Balance of the trunk | 4 |
| | | | | | Stereotyped repetitive movement of the neck | 1 |
| (4) Yagi | 7 | 4 (57.1%) | 2 (28.6%) | 1 (14.3%) | Tremor of the upper extremity | |
| | | | | | Balance | |
| Total of (1)–(4) | 63 | 36 (57.1%) 58 (92.0%) | 22 (34.9%) | 5 (7.9%) | | |
| (5) Kinoshita | 56 | 56 (100%) | 0 | | Choreatic movement of the finger | 4 |
| | | | | | Tic-like movement of the face | 1 |
| (6) Karasuyama | 32 | 32 (100%) | 0 | | Athetose-like movement | 11 |
| | | | | | Tic-like movement of the face | 1 |
| | | | | | Dystonia of the neck | 1 |
| Total of (1)–(6) | 151 | 146 (96.7%) | 5 (3.3%) | | | |

and with other people because of their apathy as a symptom of the primary mental disease, they do not seem to be aware of the manifestations of tardive dyskinesia. On the other hand, in the cases of outpatients with tardive dyskinesia, the symptoms are often enhanced by execution of daily activities, and they are often worried about abnormal movements that they or others notice.

Cole (1975) announced that there were already some suits against neuroleptic treatment causing tardive dyskinesia as the iatrogenic reaction in the United States in 1974, but we have not noted such problems in Japan. According to my experience, patients under the following conditions are often painfully aware of their abnormal dyskinetic movements: (1) schizophrenic patients who have either already recovered from psychotic symptoms completely, or are markedly improved enough to execute normal social activities but still have neuroleptic-induced tardive dyskinesia; (2) non-psychotic patients with tardive dyskinesia caused by long-term administration of antipsychotic drugs, which have been used for the purpose of, e.g., relieving neurotic anxiety, as antihypertensive drugs (such as reserpine and decaserpine), or as drugs used to treat gastric disorders (such as sulpiride and metoclopromide) and are capable of exerting influence on the extrapyramidal system.

## D.  PATIENT CHARACTERISTICS

### 1.  Sex

Many reports in Western countries indicate that female patients are more frequently affected by tardive dyskinesia than males. For example, of the four cases reported by Sigwald et al. (1959) all were females. In Degwitz's report (1966) in a sample of 672 females, tardive dyskinesia was found in 100; whereas in a sample of 619 males, 37 had the syndrome. Hunter (1964), Demars (1966), Freyhan, and Ayd (1972) also reported the prevalence in females to be higher than in males. Villeneuve states that acute dyskinesia was found twice as frequently in males, but the prevalence of tardive dyskinesia was twice as great in females. Although recent papers by some investigators report that no marked difference exists between the prevalence of tardive dyskinesia in males and females, the higher prevalence in females is still identified in Western countries. In Japan, several systematic studies on the prevalence of tardive dyskinesia have been carried out, and the prevalence ratio of male to female was 17.1 percent to 18.9 percent (Ogita et al., 1975), 7 to 3 in our first survey on severe, irreversible cases (Itoh et al., 1971, 1973), 10.3 percent to 14.8 percent (Yagi et al., 1976), and 4.8 percent to 10.9 percent (Kinoshita et al., 1973). These systematic studies showed equal prevalence in both sexes in Japan.

## 2. Age

Ayd (1967, 1972) reported that acute (early) dyskinesia was most prevalent between the ages of 5 and 45, especially in younger patients, whereas tardive dyskinesia appeared most often in patients over 50 years of age. Crane (1968) investigated 279 cases and found the average age of the patients to be in their 50s and 60s (the youngest age was 27, and the oldest age was 82). Demars (1966) stated that the average age of tardive dyskinesia was higher by nine years than that of the general inpatient population. On the other hand, Sied and Müller (1967) reported that in the geriatric wards, the age distribution of tardive dyskinesia patients was similar to that of all hospitalized patients.

The age of the dyskinetic patients in our first survey (Itoh et al., 1971) ranged from 27 to 62 years (average age, 47.3 years). The results of the cross-national comparative survey in 1972 by Ogita et al. showed that patients ranged in age from 38 to 67 years (average age, 51.5 years) at Inogashira Hospital in Japan, and from 41 to 83 years (average age, 63.8 years) at Hôpital Psychiatrique de Bassens in France. Yet another study by Yagi at Minagawa Hospital in Japan reported that the age distribution was between 29 and 72 years (average age, 47.4 years).

Summarize the above-mentioned reports, it is suggested that, under the same conditions in dosage level and duration of the given neuroleptics, the older the patient, the more likely was tardive dyskinesia to occur.

## 3. Psychiatric Disorders and Somatic Complications

There is no apparent correlation between tardive dyskinesia and the patient's original psychiatric diagnosis that has become subject for neuroleptic treatment. Most of the long-term hospitalized patients under neuroleptic treatment are schizophrenic patients. Therefore, it may be considered that shizophrenic patients are vulnerable to this syndrome. However, tardive dyskinesia may also occur in cases of chronic brain disorders, manic-depressive psychosis, and non-psychotic disorders. Two cases in the first report on this syndrome by Sigwald were under the administration of chlorpromazine for releiving neurologic pain. One third of the cases surveyed at Hôpital Psychiatrique de Bassens (France) in 1971 by Ogita and co-workers were non-schizophrenic psychiatric patients.

As for somatic complications, there exist some conflicting opinions as to whether patients with organic brain abnormalities have higher incidences of tardive dyskinesia. In Japan, the complications of cerebral arteriosclerosis or other organic brain abnormalities were identified from 50 to 68 percent by Ogita et al. (1975) Karasuyama et al. (1972), and Kinoshita et al. (1973). In Western countries, these complications were found in 15 out of 29 cases by Uhrbrand and Faurbye (1960) (including the cases whose dyskinesia was caused only by ECT or lobotomy), and in 15 patients out of 43 with tardive dyskinesia by Crane (1968).

Pryce and Edwards (1966) and Degwitz et al. (1966) described that the patient's history of organic brain abnormality did not influence the incidence of tardive dyskinesia. However, Edwards (1970) compared the incidence of brain damage and buccal abnormalities between a group of 34 elderly female chronic patients with persistent dyskinesia and a control group of 34 patients, both of which were matched in sex, age, and phenothiazine intake. He postulated that the dyskinetic group showed a significant excess in the incidence of brain damage (incident rate: 82 percent in the dyskinetic group; 41 percent in the control group).

From the results of the survey by Edwards that the occurrence rate was 44 percent in the patient group receiving ECT, and 23 percent in the group without previous ECT, Demars (1966) considered that administration of ECT influenced the incidence of tardive dyskinesia. But he found no significant correlation between tardive dyskinesia and lobotomy.

High incidence of tardive dyskinesia in the cases with organic brain abnormalities were also reported on the basis of findings utilizing pneumo-encephalographic (Hunter et al., 1964; Haddenbrock, 1966; Faurbye et al., 1964) or electroencephalographic procedures (Paulson, 1968; Sied and Müller, 1967). Kazamatsuri (1971) described that, when investigators intend to study the relationship between tardive dyskinesia and organic brain damage, they should consider that most patients receiving ECT, lobotomy, or insulin shock therapy might have suffered from severe psychotic diseases and have taken a considerable amount of antipsychotic drugs. In our previous survey, patients with history or complication of encephalitis, head injury, and generalized vascular diseases such as hypertension, arteriosclerosis, diabetes mellitus, etc., were observed far more frequently in the dyskinetic group compared with the control group.

Considering the above together with the fact that the occurrence of tardive dyskinesia is concentrated on the eldery patient's strata, it is logical to suggest—though still highly speculative—that there are etiological relations to vascular diseases involving the central nervous system.

## 4. Race

Denber et al. (1962) reported a remarkable difference in therapeutic effects and incidence of side effects of neuroleptics between Liege and New York; it was conceivable that the incidence, patient's characteristics, and clinical pictures of tardive dyskinesia would differ according to country and race.

According to the results of an investigation of 156 in-patients at Boston State Hospital and of 1,072 in-patients at 5 mental hospitals around Tokyo made by Kazamatsuri et al. (1973) and others, the incidence of serious dyskinesia in Japan is much lower than that in America. In order to find a clue to this problem, an investigation was carried out in Hôpital Psychiatrique de Bassens (France) and Inogashira Hospital (Japan) by Ogita et al. (1975). In each hospital, patients hospitalized and under psychotropic medication for more than 3 months were chosen. Presence of persistent dyskinesia in the two hospitals was checked by the same doctor on the basis of the same diagnostic criteria.

The results were presented at the IX Congress of the Collegium International Neuropsychopharmacologicum in Paris in 1974. Tardive dyskinesia was noted in 24 of 131 patients at Bassens (18.3 percent), and in 22 of 123 patients at Inogashira Hospital (17.9 percent); there was no difference in the prevalence between the two patient populations. Although various characteristics of the patients with this symptom were studied, no marked difference was seen between the two groups, but minor difference in age-sex distribution existed.

In general, cases of dyskinesia at Bassens were less intermittent and more pronounced than those at Inogashira, regardless of similarity in nature of the manifestation. Except for the relatively low incidence of rolling movement of the tongue in patients at Inogashira, a marked similarity of symptoms between the two hospitals must be stressed. Lingual dyskinesia, the most typical symptom of oral dyskinesia, was observed in all cases at Bassens, whereas at Inogashira, it was observed in only half the cases. There also existed a considerable contrast between the psychotropic medication used at the two hospitals. The daily dose of sedative neuroleptics was similar in both hospitals (chlorpromazine, 100 to 500 mg; levomepromazine, 100 to 400 mg); but these neuroleptics, alone or in combination with other neuroleptics, were in generally more frequently prescribed to chronic patients at Inogashira Hospital than at Bassens Hospital.

As for the incisive neuroleptics, a more marked difference was noted between the two hospitals. Fluphenazine was administered far more frequently, and its daily dose reached 200 to 300 mg at Bassens; whereas at Inogashira, it was seldom administered and then only at the level of 1 to 6 mg per day. Prochlorperazine and triflupromazine were also more frequently used at Bassens, and the daily doses were higher there than at Inogashira.

Injectable long-acting neuroleptics, such as fluphenazine enanthate, fluphenazine decanoate, and fluspirilene were administered to 10 out of 23 subjects exhibiting persistent dyskinesia at Bassens; whereas at Inogashira, none of the 22 subjects received these drugs. At Inogashira, perphenazine and haloperidol were administered to two thirds of the subjects at daily doses of 12 to 48 mg and 1 to 10 mg, respectively. Perphenazine and haloperidol were rarely used at Bassens. Such differences in the prescription of neuroleptics as described above seemed to be related not by prevalence but by the severity of the symptoms.

The hereditary or predisposing factors have been conceived for tardive dyskinesia to be induced by long-term neuroleptic administration. Though many of the patients have received long-term high-dosage administration of neuroleptics, only a few cases have tardive dyskinesia. A number of psychiatrists seem to have clinical experience of patients with persistent dyskinesia and/or hypertonic abnormal movements induced by short-term low-dosage neuroleptic administration, that is, as short as a few months. However, the existence of this predisposing factor has not been certified until now.

Myrianthopoulos et al. (1962) pointed out hereditary factors as the individual predisposition of neuroleptic-induced Parkinsonism, and Brandon et al. (1971) also suggested the influence of genetic factors on tardive dyskiensia from the result of high incidence of facial dyskinesia in blue-eyed men. Gardos et al. (1976) could not show the relationship between dyskinesia and eye color in a supplementary investigation, but it is a future subject to check the individual predisposing factor that causes dyskinesia.

## E.  CAUSAL PSYCHOTROPIC TREATMENT

### 1.  Causal Psychotropics

Neuroleptics are undoubtedly the main factor of this syndrome. But it is not always easy to identify the causal neuroleptics in each case for the reasons described as follows: (1) a great number of psychotropic drugs are used in daily psychiatric practice; (2) several kinds of neuroleptics are frequently prescribed concomitantly; and (3) the prescription is extremely changeable.

Uhrbrand and Faurbye (1960, 1964) described in their reports that piperazine phenothiazines (like perphenazine, thioridazine, or prochlorperazine) and haloperidol were reputed to produce the highest incidence of tardive dyskinesia. Table 3 shows the types of neuroleptics and the number of cases receiving prescribed neuroleptics for tardive dyskinesia in Japan.

Summarizing the results of the surveys in Japan, it is difficult to find definite evidence for the correlation between the manifestation of dyskinesia and a certain type of antipsychotic drugs.

From the author's impression, unlike the early drug-induced extrapyramidal symptoms (akathisia, acute dystonic reactions, and drug-induced Parkinsonism), all phenothiazines, butyrophenones, and long-acting neuroleptics (fluphenazine enanthate, fluphenazine decanoate, pimozid, fluspirilene, etc.) (Villeneuve et al., 1969; Villeneuve and Boszormenyi, 1970)—including not only incisive neuroleptics like piperazine-phenothiazines—but

Table 3. Previous Neuroleptic Treatment for the Patients with Tardive Dyskinesia

| | Name of Administered Neuroleptic* | Concomitant Use of Anti-Parkinsonian Drugs |
|---|---|---|
| Itoh | Chlorpromazine (6/10), levomepromazine (4/10), haloperidol (1/10), perazine (1/10), prochlorperazine (1/10) | 8/10 + |
| Ogita (France) | Thioproperazine, levomepromazine, thioridazine, propericiazine trifupromazine, prochlorperazine, fluphenanzine haloperidol, fluphenazine enanthate, fluphenazine decanoate, fluspirilene | 2/3 + |
| Ogita | Chlorpromazine (86.4%), perphenazine (68.2%), haloperidol (63.6%), levomepromazine (54.5%), thioridazine (50.0%), fluphenazine (36.4%), propericiazine (27.3%), chlorprothixene (2/22), carpipramine (2/22), triperidol (2/22), prochlcrperazine (2/22), perazine (2/22), spiclomazine (1/22), clothiapine (1/22), thioproperazine (1/22), reserpine (1/22), thiothixene (1/22) | 13/22 + |
| Yagi | Levomepromazine (2/7), perazine (3/7), thioproperazine (1/7), chlorpromazine (1/7), perphenazine (1/7), haloperidol (1/7), thiothixene (1/7 | |
| Kinoshita | Chlorpromazine (54%), haloperidol (14%), perphenazine (9%), imipramine (2/56), amitriptyline (1/56) | |

*Number of administered cases/total number of patients with tardive dyskinesia).

also sedative neuroleptics, such as chlorpromazine and levomepromazine, are able to become responsible agents. Furthermore, we have observed cases of tardive dyskinesia that were apparently caused by the use of reserpine and tetrabenazine, both belonging to dopamine-releasing agents, and by some neuroleptics with different types of chemical structures, such as clothiapine, carpipramine, and oxypertine.

There are also some reports showing that orofacial dyskinesia or choreiform syndrome, though uncommon, occurred by the use of some psychotropics other than neuroleptics, such as tricyclic antidepressants, anticholinergic anti-parkinsonian drugs (trihexyphenidyl), phenytoin, amphetamine, and others.

The author has studied a few cases of persistent dyskinesia, which manifested after sudden withdrawal of long-term treatment with non-psychotropic drugs, such as rauwolfia alkaloids, given as the anti-hypertensive agent, or sulpiride and metoclopramide for stomach diseases. These dyskinetic movements, so-called withdrawal dyskinesia, continued for a few months or years.

## 2. Dosage and Duration of Causal Drugs

As for the dosage and duration of responsible neuroleptics, long-term medication and a great amount of it seemed to cause tardive dyskinesia most frequently, but no precise evidence supports these impressions because of difficulties in identifying the date of onset and frequent changes of prescription or combined use of neuroleptics in many of the patients with tardive dyskinesia. Among 17 cases reported by us, the number receiving long-term high-dosage neuroleptic treatment was few. All three cases reported by Karasuyama et al. (1972) were also given low or medium dosage phenothiazines for 2 to 4 years.

According to Ogita's report, the ordinal daily doses of incisive neuroliptics at Hôpital Psychiatrique de Bassens (France) were several times higher than those at Inogashira Hospital (Japan). For example, daily doses of fluphenazine reached 200 to 300 mg at Bassens, whereas at Inogashira, doses only reached the level of 1 to 6 mg a day; and the average single dose of fluphenazine every 2 weeks was 100 mg at Bassens and 25 mg at Inogashira. Nevertheless, no difference was observed in prevalence at these hospitals.

Ayd (1967) stated that the average period from the beginning of psychotropic treatment to the onset of persistent dyskinesia was about 24 months. Haddenbrock (1966) reported that one case of persistent dyskinesia appeared after administration of perphenazine at a dose of 70 mg per day for 3 months; that was the representative case of tardive dyskinesia developing after the shortest period of neuroleptic administration.

The period of neuroleptic treatment necessary for inducing tardive dyskinesia ranges widely from a few months to years according to both our clinical experiences and the literature. There are many reports stating that the high incidence of dyskinesia was shown in patients who received high-dose neuroleptic therapy or a large amount in total. However, high-dose long-term use of psychotropic drugs does not always cause tardive dyskinesia, because not only such external variables as the type, dose, and administration period of drugs influence the manifestation of the syndrome, but also the patient's individual factors. But individually, it may be considered that the possibility of tardive dyskinesia increases with the prolongation of high-dose psychotropic therapy.

A few investigators indicated that treatment with anti-parkinsonian agents or tricyclic antidepressants increased the patient's risk of having tardive dyskinesia (Fann, 1972, 1974).

## F.  DIFFERENTIAL DIAGNOSIS

The diagnosis of tardive dyskinesia is generally easy. When persistent, stereotyped and repetitive movements occur around the mouth of the patient who has received psychotropic drug treatment for a long time, and it can be diagnose as tardive dyskinesia (Kazamatsuri, 1971). The diseases to be differentiated from tardive dyskinesia are as follows:

Parkinson's disease
Drug-induced Parkinsonism
Drug-induced acute dystonic reactions
Huntington's chorea
Syndenham's chorea
Dementia paralytica
Hepatolenticular degeneration
Levodopa-induced dyskinesia
Psychotic posturing, stereotypy, etc.
Dystonia musculorum deformans
Spontaneous senile tremor, or BLM syndrome
Others (hemiballisms, torticallis)

According to clinical experience, it is not difficult to distinguish tardive dyskinesia from the above disorders, which manifest similar abnormal movements, if the characteristics previously described in the section, "Clinical Features and Localization" and the most recent psychotropic drug treatments are taken into consideration. However, differentiation between tardive dyskinesia and spontaneous senile bucco-linguo-masticatory dyskinesia or tremor, which occurs with no medication and is discovered in a small percentage of the patients hospitalized in geriatric wards, is difficult only through clinical observation of its symptomatology. And extremely slight tardive dyskinesia is likely to be misdiagnosed as stereotyped autistic movements of psychotic symptom.

The relation of tardive dyskinesia to other drug-induced extrapyramidal symptoms, levodopa-induced dyskinesia, and Huntington's chorea will be described in the following sections.

## G. RELATIONSHIP BETWEEN TARDIVE DYSKINESIA AND OTHER DRUG-INDUCED EXTRAPYRAMIDAL SYMPTOMS

Table 4 shows the different characteristics of tardive dyskinesia from those of other drug-induced extrapyramidal symptoms.

Differential diagnosis among tardive dyskinesia and other drug-induced extrapyramidal reactions can be made from consideration of the onset, affected portion, clinical course, influence of drug removal, effect of anti-Parkinsonian agents, and so on. The patients with akathisia and acute dyskinesia complain of anxiety, irritability, distress, or disability in daily activities; whereas, in the case of tardive dyskinesia, such psychiatric and subjective symptoms are seldom observed. According to Freyhan, the percentages of Parkinsonism, which developed after the commencement of administration of chlorpromazine and reserpine, were 62.0 and 51.7 percent, respectively in the period within 30 days, 22.5 and 27.6 percent within 30 to 60 days, 11.2 and percent within 61 to 90 days, and 4.7 and 20.7 percent after 91 days. That is, 38.0 to 48.3 percent of Parkinsonism developed within 1 month after the administration, and 4.3 to 20.7 percent manifested 3 months later.

The statistical results of the survey by Ayd showed that cumulative percentage of the occurrence of Parkinsonism and akathisia reached 90 percent about $2\frac{1}{2}$ months later, and the remaining 10 percent developed thereafter. Therefore, considering "syndrome précoces" observed immediately after administration and "syndrome intermédiaires" (Wertheimer, 1968) observed a few months later, the onset of tardive dyskinesia and other drug-induced extrapyramidal symptoms broadly overlap one another. As for the characteristics of the symptoms, there is a considerable resemblance between early dyskinesia and tardive dyskinesia in the body areas and the features of abnormal movements.

Rabbit syndrome advocated by Villeneuve (1972) (perioral muscular movements strikingly imitating the rapid, chewing-like movements of the rabbit's mouth) is the transitional form of both types of dyskinesia and is often successfully controlled with anti-Parkinsonian medication.

Furthermore, co-existence of tardive dyskinesia with other types of drug-induced extrapyramidal symptoms is not rare. In making diagnosis of tardive dyskinesia, careful attention should be paid to this problem.

Table 4. Characteristics of Drug-Induced Extra-Pyramidal Symptoms

| | Parkinsonism | Akathisia | Dyskinesia | Tardive Dyskinesia |
|---|---|---|---|---|
| Incidence | 15.4*<br>37.3** | 21.2*<br>46.0** | 2.3*<br>8.0** | 10–30 (Overseas)<br>5–20 (Japan) |
| Sex | 1(Male):2(Female) | 1(Male):2(Female) | 2(Male):1(Female) | Male Female (Overseas)<br>Male Female (Japan) |
| Age | Senile | Mid-Age | Juvenile | Senile |
| Drug liable to cause symptoms | Phenothiazine of piperazine group, butyrophenone | | | No particular drug (?) |
| Time of onset | Usually after 2 weeks | Usually after 1 week | After 1–3 days, or after a sharp increase in dosage | Usually after 1-year period (?) |
| Site of onset | Generalized | Restless legs | Eyes, mouth, tongue, neck, chin, trunk, extremities | Chiefly in mouth, tongue, and chin (expanding to neck, trunk, and extremities on some occasions) |
| Progress | Prolonged | Severity changes | Transient (rarely lasting over 24 hours) | Prolonged |
| Effect of anti-Parkinsonism drugs | Good | Good | Good | Poor |
| Psychotic symptoms | Depression | Anxiety, impatience, depression | Anxiety, impatience, enhanced suggestibility | No particular symptoms |

* Denotes results of investigation on 3,775 patients on phenothiazine (by F. Ayd). No such clear tendency of sex and age was noted in a survey made by Tsuji.
** Denotes results of investigation on 150 patients on butyrophenone (by E. Tsuji).

## H. RELATIONSHIP BETWEEN TARDIVE DYSKINESIA, LEVODOPA-INDUCED DYSKINESIA, AND HUNTINGTON'S CHOREA

With respect to the symptomatology and response to various kinds of drugs, tardive dyskinesia is very similar to levodopa-induced dyskinesia and Huntington's chorea. Although the etiology is different in the three disorders, the basic mechanisms may closely resemble one another. So, the comparison between the disorders is not only interesting but also important for studying other neurological disorders with unknown etiology. Table 5 shows the clinical-pharmacological comparison among the three disorders.

Neurological symptoms are all represented by stereotyped dyskinetic movements, particularly BLM syndrome, though the etiology or responsible drugs are different. The abnormal movements of Huntington's chorea are described as playful movements mixed with slight normal motions and appear more prominently in the proximal parts of the limbs than in the perioral area.

Levodopa-induced dyskinesia worsens as the amount of levodopa is increased and improves or disappears by reduction in dose. Tardive dyskinesia and Huntington's chorea are also aggravated with the administration of levodopa.

Dyskinetic movements of levodopa-induced dyskinesia and Huntington's chorea certainly mitigate with the administration of dopamine-blocking agents, such as phenothiazines and butyrophenones, but Parkinsonism is enhanced. In tardive dyskinesia, dyskinetic movements may be worsened transiently or remain unchanged by reduction or discontinuation of responsible neuroleptics, but the symptoms are often ameliorated only by the long-term removal of causal antipsychotic drugs. On the other hand, tardive dyskinesia is mitigated by increasing neuroleptics, but, is exacerbated and progresses gradually if the situation is continued over a long period.

Similar tendency is also observed in levodopa-induced dyskinesia and Huntington's chorea. When dopamine-depleting agents such as reserpine and tetrabenazine are given, the same results can be obtained as when dopamine-blockung agents are administered in these three conditions.

Each dyskinesia remains unchanged or progresses with the administration of anticholinergic agents. As for the clinical course, levodopa-induced dyskinesia improves or disappears by reduction of levodopa, but Parkinsonism worsens. The author confirms the fact that tardive dyskinesia improved or disappeared gradually during the long-term clinical course by withdrawing neuroleptics at an early stage, but in many cases, the patient's psychopathology may be aggravated during neuroleptic removal. The dilemma like

**Table 5. Clinical Features and Effects of Various Agents in Tardive Dyskinesia, Levodopa-Induced Dyskinesia, and Huntington's Chorea**

| | Tardive Dyskinesia | Levodopa-Induced Dyskinesia | Huntington's Chorea |
|---|---|---|---|
| Responsible medication | Long-term administration or abrupt withdrawal of drugs with striatal potency (mainly, neuroleptics) | Administration of levolopa | None |
| Neurological symptoms | Stereotyped dyskinetic movements, particularly BLM syndrome | Stereotyped dyskinetic movements, particularly BLM syndrome | Stereotyped dyskinetic movements, but playful movements appear more in the limbs |
| Levodopa | aggravated | Aggravated when dosage increased, improved or disappeared when dosage reduced | Aggravate |
| Dopamine-blocking agents (phenothiazines, butyrophenones) | Dosage increase–transiently improved, but enhanced after long-term medication<br><br>Dosage reduction or discontinuation—transiently aggravated, but gradually ameliorated | Improved, but Parkinsonism enhanced | Improved, but aggravated again after long-term medication |

## Table 5. (continued)

| | Tardive Dyskinesia | Levodopa-Induced Dyskinesia | Huntington's Chorea |
|---|---|---|---|
| Dopamine-depleting agents (reserpine, tetrabenazine) | Improved, but Parkinsonism may appear; aggravated again after long-term medication | Improved, but Parkinsonism may appear; aggravated again after long-term medication | Improved, but Parkinsonism may appear; aggravated again after long-term medication |
| Anti-cholinergic agents | Unchanged or aggravated | Unchanged or aggravated | Unchanged or aggravated |
| Physostigmine | Improved | Improved | Improved |
| Clinical course | Sometimes irreversible | Reversible | Irreversible, but changeable during long-term period |
| Dilemma in executing therapy | Neuroleptic discontinuation—dyskinesia improved, psychotic symptoms exacerbated | Levodopa discontinuation—dyskinesia improved, Parkinsonism worsened | |

these phenomena is so-called "the dilemma of the therapy", which is becoming a perplexing problem in daily clinical practice.

## I. REVERSIBILITY OF TARDIVE DYSKINESIA

Unlike the early drug-induced extrapyramidal symptoms, such as Parkinsonism and acute dystonic reaction, tardive dyskinesia persists for years despite discontinuation of antipsychotic drugs. Therefore, tardive dyskinesia is also called "persistent dyskinesia," "terminal extrapyramidal insufficiency," and even "irreversible dyskinesia."

Literature indicates that, in the majority of patients, dyskinesia can be permanent or irreversible. On the other hand, some investigators suggest that the earlier the dyskinesia is detected and the responsible neuroleptic stopped, the better is the prognosis for amelioration (Ayd, 1976; Crane, 1975; Curran, 1973; Donlon and Stenson, 1976; Quitkin et al., 1977). According to opinion of these authors, it is not always true that the terms "tardive dyskinesia" and "irreversible dyskinesia" are interchangeable. Today, the opinions on the natural course of this syndrome are still confused. Many psychiatrists and neurologists having patients with tardive dyskinesia are likely to consider the syndrome irreversible. Actually, one case with tardive dyskinesia was described as lasting for 14 years.

The earlier report by Uhrbrand and Faurbye (1960), in which the term "irreversible dyskinesia" was probably used for the first time, stated that, in 11 of 17 cases in which antipsychotic treatment was discontinued, dyskinesia proved irreversible after an observation period of 4 to 22 months.

Recently, some investigators pointed out that long-term observation after complete cessation of the neuroleptic treatment would be necessary for determining whether dyskinesia was reversible or irreversible. In a follow-up investigation, the authors made a long-term study of patients with tardive dyskinesia, where neuroleptic treatment had been discontinued for as long as 5 years, from 1971 to 1976. This study suggested that: (1) in many of the patients with tardive dyskinesia, the symptoms can be considerably improved only with neuroleptic withdrawal, and (2) the pharmacological treatment of tardive dyskinesia could become material for discussion in view of long-term prognosis of the syndrome (especially that the administration of certain neuroleptics only for the treatment of dyskinesia is inappropriate).

In 1971, through a simultaneous total survey of abnormal involuntary movements, we found 19 patients with severe tardive dyskinesia in 7 hospitals. At the time of the survey, dyskinesia was judged irreversible, because reduction or discontinuation of neuroleptics executed several months or years before had produced no change. To follow up the symptomatology of these 19 cases for 5 years, the Abnormal Involuntary Movement Scale (AIMS) by NIMH (NIMH, 1975) and the video- or movie-recording technique developed by our research group were used (Itoh et al., 1976; Itoh and Yagi, 1977). Though the symptoms persisted in all of the patients, ameliorations in various grades took place in the majority of them, and progressive aggravation was not observed.

Marked ameliorations of dyskinetic symptoms were observed in the younger group, while the persistence of abnormal movements judged "unchanged" was found only in the elderly group. It should be noted that, in the group of patients under age 60, amelioration was achieved in 100 percent of the cases.

As a result of the long-term follow-up study for 5 years, marked and moderate amelioration was observed in the majority of patients with long-term dyskinesia persisting over 8 years, whereas slight amelioration and unchanged cases were observed in half of the patients with rather short-term persisting dyskinesia.

With concomitant use of this video- and/or movie-recording technique and assessment with AIMS in accordance with the standardized examination procedure, a more advanced, more systematic, and more objective follow-up study on tardive dyskinesia could be established. Since it has already been pointed out that the judgment of tardive dyskinesia should be carried out after neuroleptic withdrawal, the fact that in the present study, some of our subjects received neuroleptics intermittently during the follow-up period, may certainly be questioned. But neuroleptics were given at low doses and no remarkable tendency of improvement was shown in these patients. In those cases whose psychotic symptoms persisted, clinical judgment on tardive dyskinesia under the neuroleptic continuation was inevitable.

The fact that in some cases, tardive dyskinesia disappears or is relieved, whereas in other cases, there is a worsening of dyskinetic movements after discontinuance of neuroleptics, was already pointed out by Faurbye et al. (1964), Haddenbrock (1966), Degwitz et al. (1967), Edwards (1970), Crane (1975), Turunen and Achté (1967), and Curran (1973).

We have already shown that in the natural course of tardive dyskinesia, "persistent" does not always mean "irreversible" (Itoh et al., 1973, 1976; Itoh and Yagi, 1977). Previously, it was reported that in young adults, persistent dyskinesia had disappeared within several weeks or months by early removal of the drugs (Yagi et al., 1976). Otani et al. (1974) and Moline (1975) also reported reversible dyskinesia among younger patients.

In our report, using a movie-recording technique, we demonstrated that one elderly patient, who received neuroleptics for several years and had fully developed dyskinetic movements, could be cleared of dyskinesia completely with long-term neuroleptic withdrawal. This evidence urges us to correct the belief that tardive dyskinesia is irreversible.

It is a well-known fact that the patient's age plays an important role in the appearance of tardive dyskinesia. In the present study, age seemed to be an important contributing factor to the possibility of amelioration of long-lasting dyskinesia after discontinuation of drugs. In younger patients, considerable improvement could be expected; while in the elderly group, the more advanced the patient's age, the more marked was the tendency to remain in an unchanged condition. In this respect, a follow-up study on an elderly group might show a lower amelioration rate. In the early stages after neuroleptic withdrawal, there were a variety of clinical courses where patients exhibited not only improvement but also transient worsening. But after that, gradual reduction in symptomatology was observed in the majority of cases following long-term removal of drugs. These characteristics in the clinical course of tardive dyskinesia should be taken into consideration when biochemical aspects of pharmacology of the symptoms are discussed (Donlon and Stenson, 1976; Fann et al., 1977; Klawans, 1973; Klawans and Rubovits, 1975; Seeman et al., 1974).

Since the beginning of 1970, a variety of pharmacological treatments, based on biochemical hypotheses for tardive dyskinesia have been actively tried, and it has been reported that many drugs seemed to have been effective in relieving this condition (Ayd, 1972; Gardos et al., 1977; Kazamatsuri et al., 1972). But the evaluation of these effects was made by short-term clinical observation within a few weeks or months, and furthermore in the practice of many of these evasive therapeutic drugs, dyskinetic symptoms have reappeared soon after interrruption of the medication. Therefore the pharmacological treatments for tardive dyskinesia are at present extremely unsatisfactory, and care should be taken to prevent untoward influences on the long-term prognosis of tardive dyskinesia. It seems that administration of certain neuroleptics only for the treatment of tardive dyskinesia is inappropriate. As pointed out by some investigators, prolonged administration of neuroleptics, which possess dopamine-blocking or dopamine-releasing action, causes hypersensitivity of striatal dopamine-facilitated receptors and even structural changes, and consequently dyskinesia becomes permanent.

Schiele (1976) and Tuason (1976) emphasized that no medication, including removal of causative neuroleptics, was the best treatment for tardive dyskinesia at present. The results obtained from our present study support their opinions to some extent. Though complete neuroleptic withdrawal is the most desirable method of preventing tardive dyskinesia from becoming irreversible, prolonged discontinuation of neuroleptic therapy over a few years, especially in schizophrenic patients, is frequently difficult because of persistence, worsening, or recurrence of psychotic symptoms.

In this investigation, many patients had to receive certain neuroleptics intermittently during a period of 5 years. Further research is needed to establish the appropriate drug therapy for psychotic states of schizophrenic patients with tardive dyskinesia and to make clear the influences of inter-mittent neuroleptic therapy, which is carried out for the management of transient worsening or recurrence of psychotic conditions, in the long-term prognosis of tardive dyskinesia.

## J.  TREATMENTS AND PROPHYLAXIS OF TARDIVE DYSKINESIA

When tardive dyskinesia occurs, neuroleptic administration should be stopped as much as possible. If the drug removal is carried out in the early stages of tardive dyskinesia, most symptoms imporve or disappear within a few weeks or months. Even in cases of long-lasting persistent dyskinesia, it is common for a patient to recover almost completely within a few years through drug withdrawal. However, when the drug withdrawal worsens patient's psychiatric condition, the administration of neuroleptics should be continued. In these cases, it is recommended that neuroleptics with low striatal potency be used as much as possible (for example, thioridazine, pipanperon, and others). Sometimes, involuntary movements are enhanced temporarily by drug removal, but mitigate thereafter.

The therapist should consider his therapeutic policy not only to control dyskinesia immediately, but also to make the long-term prognosis favorable.

Dopamine-blocking agents, such as phenothiazines and butyrophe-nones were once used on a trial basis to control involuntary movements (Kazamatsuri et al., 1973). As a result, these drugs control the movements temporarily, but soon make them worse so they require more administra-tion, and finally, dyskinetic movements become irreversible. Therefore, the use of these types of drugs cannot be recommended.

There are some reports mentioning that the administration of dopamine-depleting agents (reserpine, tetrabenazine, etc.) and oxypertine may alleviate the symptoms, but, on the contrary, we experienced dyskinetic cases caused by these drugs. It was also reported that clozapine was effective against both tardive dyskinesia and psychiatric symptoms (Simpson et al., 1978), but this drug often produces serious secondary reactions with fever and agranulocytosis. In addition, clinical experiences in using blocker of catecholamine synthesis ($\alpha$-methyldopa, $\alpha$-methylparathyrosine) (Ville-neuve, 1970; Tzavellas et al., 1967; Gerlach and Thorsen, 1976; Gerlach, 1977), blocker of catecholamine release (lithium salts) (Simpson et al., 1978), cholinergic agents (deanol, physostigmine) (Bochenheimer and Lucius, 1976; Casey and Denney, 1975, 1977; Simpson and Kline, 1976; Stafford et al., 1977; Tamminga et al., 1977; Davis et al., 1976), and GABA-related agents (sodium valproate, baclofen) were reported (Ayd, 1976; Gerlach, 1977; Gerlach et al., 1978; Korsgaard, 1976), but the sufficient efficacy of these drugs has not been evaluated up to the present. The effect of stereotactic surgical operation has not yet been sufficiently evaluated either. The early diagnosis and the early removal of causal drugs are desirable for tardive dyskinesia (Crane, 1977), and the preventive measures are as follows:

1. Neuroleptic administration in an unnecessarily large amount to long-term treated patients should be avoided, and the maintenance dose should be minimized as much as possible.
2. If initial signs of tardive dyskinesia (fine vermicular involuntary movements of the tongue and/or lips) are observed, the administration of responsible drugs (mainly neuroleptics) should be stopped.
3. Careful attention should be paid to the treatment of elderly patients.
4. Long-term concomitant use of anti-Parkinsonian agents should be avoided.
5. The trial of providing drug holiday may be advocated.

## K. CONCLUSION

Although tardive dyskinesia is the associated symptom based on the pharmacological action of neuroleptics, it is an obvious iatrogenic neurological distrubance and an incurable extrapyramidal disorder that were caused by long-term neuroleptic administration for the treatment of psychiatric disorders.

Tardive dyskinesia occurred in 5 to 20 percent of hospitalized chronic psychotic patients receiving antipsychotic drug treatments in Japan. This fact suggests that the manifestation of tardive dyskinesia will become a serious problem in the investigation of psychotropic drug treatment.

Up to the present, various treatments have been investigated, based on the neuropharmacological hypothesis about the etiology of tardive dyskinesia, but no successful therapy has been found among them. Nowadays, the earlier diagnosis of dyskinetic symptoms, possible withdrawal of responsible drugs, and preventive care for daily psychotropic drug treatments are regarded as extremely important for the management of this syndrome.

This chapter also referred to the symptomatology, prognosis, and management of the syndrome in order to review the guidelines for preventing the manifestation of drug-induced tardive dyskinesia.

## ACKNOWLEDGMENTS

This work was supported in part by Japanese Ministry of Education Grant No. 448248. The author wishes to thank the staff of the Clinical Psychopharmacology Research Group, Department of Neuropsychiatry, Keio University for their continuing cooperation. I am particularly grateful to J. Levine of N.I.M.H. (U.S.A.), and P. Lambert, of Hôpital Psychiatrique de Bassens (France) for their cross-national cooperation and valuable advice. Thanks are also due to Miss Kurihara and Miss Fujimura for preparing the manuscript.

## L. REFERENCES

(ACNP—FDA) American College of Neuropsychopharmacology—Food and Drug Administration Task Force (1973). Neurological syndromes associated with antipsychotic drug use. *Arch. Gen. Psychiat.* 28:463–467.

Allen, R.E., and Stimmel, G.L. (1977). Neuroleptic dosage, duration, and tardive dyskinesia. *Dis. Nerv. Syst.* 38:385–387.

Ayd, F.J., Jr. (1976a). On the reversibility of tardive dyskinesia. *Int. Drug Ther. Newsletter.* 11:9:35–36.

Ayd, F.J., Jr. (1976b). Sodium valproate therapy for tardive dyskinesia. *Int. Drug Ther. Newsletter.* 12:8, 9:29–34.

Ayd, F.J., Jr. (1972). Treatment of persistent dyskinesia. *Int. Drug Ther. Newsletter.* 7:3:9–11.

Ayd, F.J., Jr. (1967). Persistent dyskinesia: A neurological complication of major tranquilizers. *Med. Sci.* 18:32–40.

Bockenheimer, S., and Lucius, G. (1976). Zur Therapie mit Dimethylaminoethanol (Deanol) bei neuroleptika-induzierten extrapyramidalen Hyperkinesen. *Arch. Psychiat. Nervenkrank.* 222:69–75.

Bourgeois, M. (1977). Les dyskinesies tardives des neuroléptiques. Enguête chez 3,140 malades d'hôpital psychiatrique. *L'Encéphale.* 3:299–320.

Brandon, S., McClelland, H.A., and Protheroe, C. (1971). A study of facial dyskinesia in a mental hospital population. *Brit. J. Psychiat.* 118:171–184.

Casey, D.E. (1977). Deanol in the management of involuntary movement disorders: A review. *Dis. Nerv. Syst.* 38:12:2:7–15.

Casey, D.E., and Denney, D. (1977). Original investigations: Pharmacological characterization of tardive dyskinesia. *Psychopharmacol.* 54:1–8.

Casey, D.E., and Denney, D. (1975). Deanol in the treatment of tardive dyskinesia. *Am. J. Psychiat.* 132:864–867.

Chadwick, D., Reynolds, E.H., and Marsden, C.D. (1976). Anticonvulsant-induced dyskinesias: A comparison with dyskinesia induced by neuroleptics. *J. Neurol. Neurosurg. Psychiat.* 39:1210–1218.

Cole, J.O. (1975). Tardive dyskinesia—Legal and therapeutic aspects, in *Neuropsychopharmacology.* Proceedings of the IX Congress of the Collegium Internationale Neuropsychopharmacologicum, Paris, 7-12 July, 1974. J.R. Boissier, H. Hippius, and P. Pichot, eds. Excerpta Medica American Elsevier, New York. pp. 365–371.

Crane, G.E. (1977). The prevention of tardive dyskinesia. *Am. J. Psychiat.* 134:756–758.

Crane, G.E. (1975). Tardive dyskinesia: A review, in *Neuropsychopharmacology.* Proceedings of the IX Congress of the Collegium Internationale Neuropsychopharmacologicum, Paris, 7-12 July, 1974. J.R. Boissier, H. Hippius, and P. Pichot, eds. Excerpta Medica American Elsevier, New York, pp. 346–354.

Crane, G.E. (1973). Persistent dyskinesia. *Brit. J Psychiat.* 122:395–405.

Crane, G.E. (1972). Pseudoparkinsonism and tardive dyskinesia. *Arch. Neurol.* 27:426–430.

Crane, G.E. (1968a). Tardive dyskinesia in patients treated with major neuroleptics: A review of the literature. *Am. J. Psychiat.* Supp. 124:8:40–54.

Crane, G.E. (1968b). Tardive dyskinesia in schizophrenic patients treated with psychotropic drugs. *Aggressologie.* 9:209–218.

Crane, G.E., and Chase, C. (1970). High doses of trifluperazine and tradive dyskinesia. *Arch. Neurol.* 22:176-180.

Crane, G.E., and Paulson, G. (1967). Involuntary movements in a sample of chronic mental patients and their relation to the treatment with neuroleptics. *Int. J. Neuropsychiat.* 3:286-291.

Curran, J.P. (1973). Tardive dyskinesia: Side effect or not? *Am. J. Psychiat.* 130:406-410.

Curzon, G. (1968). The biochemistry of dyskinesia. *Int. Rev. Neurobiol.* 10:323-370.

Davis, K.L., Hollister, L.E., Barchas, J.D., and Berger, P.A. (1976). Cholnie in tardive dyskinesia and Huntington's disease. *Life Sci.* 19:1507-1516.

Degwitz, R., and Winzel, W. (1967). Persistent extrapyramidal side effects after long-term application of neuroleptics, in *Neuropsychopharmacology*, Vol. 5. H. Brill et al., eds. Excerpta Medica, Amsterdam. pp. 608-615.

Degwitz, R., Binsack, K.F., Herkert, H., Luxemburger, O., and Winzel, W. (1967). Zum Problem der persistierenden extrapyramidalen Hyperkinesen nach langfristiger Anwendung von Neuroleptika. *Nervenarzt.* 38:170-174.

Degwitz, R., Winzel, W., Binsack, K.F., Herkert, H., and Luxemburger, H. (1966). Zum Problem der terminalen extrapyramidalen Hyperkinesen an Hand von 1,600 langfristig mit Neuroleptika Behandelten. *Arzneimittelforsch.* 16:276-278.

Demars, J.C.A. (1966). Neuromuscular effects of long-term phenothiazine medication, ECT, and leucotomy. *J. Nerv. Ment. Dis.* 143:73-79.

Denber, H.C.B., Bente, D., and Rajjotte, P. (1962). Comparative analysis of the action of butyrylperazine of Manhattan State Hospital and the University Psychiatric Clinic at Erlangen. *Am. J. Psychiat.* 119:203-207.

De Silva, and Juang, C.Y. (1975). Deanol in tardive dyskinesia. *Brit. Med. J.* 3:466.

Donlon, P.T., and Stenson, R.L. (1976). Neuroleptic induced extrapyramidal symptoms. *Dis. Ner. Sys.* 37:629-635.

Dynes, J.B. (1970). Oral dyskinesia, occurrence, and treatment. *Dis. Nerv. Syst.* 31:854-859.

Eckman, F. (1968). Zur Problematik von Dauerschaden nach neuroleptischer Langzeitbehandlung der Gegenwart, 107:316-323.

Edwards, H. (1970). The significance of brain damage in persistent oral dyskinesia. *Brit. J. Psychiat.* 116:271-275.

Ettinger, M., and Curran, J.P. (1970). Liver disease and phenothiazines. *Minn. Med.* 53:731-736.

Ey, H., and Rappard, P. (1956). Les réactions d'intolérance vis-à-vis de la chlorpromazine. *L'Encéphale.* 45:790-796.

Fann, W.E., and Lake, C.R. (1974). On the coexistence of Parkinsonism and tardive dyskinesia. *Dis. Nerv. Syst.* 35:324-326.

Fann, W.E., Davis, J.M., and Janowsky, D.S. (1972). The prevalence of tardive dyskinesias in mental hospital patients. *Dis. Nerv. Sys.* 33:182-186.

Fann, W.E., Stafford, J.R., Malone, R.L., Frost, J.D., and Richman, B.W. (1977). Clinical research techniques in tardive dyskinesia. *Am. J. Psychiat.* 134:759-762.

Faurbye, A., Rasch, P.J., Petersen, P.B., Brandborg, G., and Pakkenberg, H. (1964). Neurological symptoms in pharmacotherapy of psychoses. *Act Psychiat. Scand.* 40:10-27.

Gardos, G., Cole, J.O., and La Brie, R. (1977). The assessment of tardive dyskinesia. *Arch. Gen. Psychiat.* 34:1206-1212.

Gardos, G., Sokal, N., Cole, J.O., and Sniffin, C. (In press). Eye color and tardive dyskinesia.

Gerlach, J. (1977). The relationship between Parkinsonism and tardive dyskinesia. *Am. J. Psychiat.* 134:781-784.

Gerlach, J., and Thorsen, K. (1976). The movement pattern of oral dyskinesia in relation to anticholinergic and antidopaminergic treatment. *Int. Pharmacopsychiat.* 11:1-7.

Gerlach, J., Rye, T., and Kristijasen, P. (1978). Effect of beclofen on tardive dyskinesia. *Psychopharmacol.* 56:145-151.

Greenblatt, D.L., Stotsky, B.A., and Di Mascio, A. (1968). Phenothiazine-induced dyskinesias in nursing home. *J. Am. Geriat. Soc.* 16:27–34.

Haddenbrock, S. (1966). Zur Wirkungsweise und zur Frage zentralorganischer Spätschäden der neuroleptischen Dauerbehandlung. *Nervenarzt.* 37:199–203.

Heinrich, K., Weckner, I., and Bender, H.J. (1968). Späte extrapyramidale Hyperkinesen bei neuroleptischer Langzeit-therapie. *Pharmacopsychiat. Neuro Psychopharmacol.* 1:169–195.

Hippius, V.H., and Lange, J. (1970). Zur Problematik der späten extrapyramidalen Hyperkinesen nach langfristiger neuroleptischer Therapie. *Arzneimittel Forsch.* 20:888–890.

Hoff, H., and Hoffman, G. (1967). Das persistierende extrapyramidale Syndrom bei neuroleptika Therapie. *Wiener Med. Wochen.* 117:14–17.

Hunter, R., Blackwood, W., Smith, M.C., and Cumings, J.N. (1968). Neuropathological findings in three cases of persistent dyskinesia following phenothiazine medication. *J. Neurolog. Sci.* 7:263–273.

Hunter, R., Earl, C.J., and Thornicroft, S. (1964). An apparent irreversible syndrome of abnormal movements following phenothiazine medication. *Proc. Roy. Soc. Med.* 57:758–762.

Itoh, H. (1977). A cross-national clinical investigation on drug-induced tardive dyskinesia. Annual Meeting of the Chinese Neuropsychiatry Association, Taipei, Nov. 12.

Itoh, H., and Yagi, G. (1977). Reversibility of tardive dyskinesia—a follow-up study and film presentation. Symposium on Tardive Dyskinesia, VI World Congress of Psychiatry, Honolulu, Aug. 29.

Itoh, H., and Yagi, G. (1976). Movies on tardive dyskinesia. Symposium on Tardive Dyskinesia. Sponsored by Hennepin County Psychiatric Society, and Minnesota Psychiatric Society, Minneapolis, June 30.

Itoh, H., Miura, S., and Yagi, G. (1976a). A method for explaining dyskinetic movements. A film presentation. *Psychopharmacolog. Bull.* 12:3–4.

Itoh, H., Miura, S., Yagi, G., et al. (1971). Irreversible dyskinesia associated with long-term usage of psychotropic drugs. *Ann. Rep. Pharmacopsychiat. Res. Found.* 3:190–195.

Itoh, H., Yagi, G., Ogita, K., Ohtsuka, N., and Miura, S. (1976b). On the reversibility of tardive dyskinesia—a follow-up study and a film presentation. X Collegium Internationale Neuropsychopharmacologicum, Quebec, July 4–9.

Itoh, H., Yagi, G., Ogita, K., and Miura, S. (1973). Irreversible dyskinesia after long-term psychopharmacotherapy. *Nippon-Ijishinpoh.* 2582:29–34.

Karasuyama, N., Fujii, K., and Takahashi, R. (1972). Tardive dyskinesia. *Clin. Neurol.* 12:678.

Kazamatsuri, H. (1971). Tardive dyskinesia—Studies in foreign countries. *Seishin Igaku.* 13:840–855.

Kazamatsuri, H., Chien, C.P., and Cole, J.O. (1973a). Long-term treatment of tardive dyskinesia with haloperiodol and tetrabenazine. *Am. J. Psychiat.* 130:479–482.

Kazamatsuri, H., Chien, C.P., and Cole, J.O. (1972a). Therapeutic approaches to tardive dyskinesia, a review of the literature. *Arch. Gen. Psychiat.* 27:491–499.

Kazamatsuri, H., Chien, C.P., and Cole, J.O. (1972b). Treatment of tardive dyskinesia (I), (II), (III). *Arch. Gen. Psych.* 27:95–99, 100–103, 824–827.

Kazamatsuri, H., Matsushita, M., and Takemura, M. (1973b). Clinical studies on tardive dyskinesia (I)—Prevalence and classification. *Ann. Rep. Pharmacother. Res. Found.* 5:201–204.

Kennedy, P.F., Hershon, H.I., and Mc Guire, R.J. (1971). Extrapyramidal disorders after prolonged phenothiazine therapy. *Brit. J. Psychiat.* 118:509–518.

Kinoshita, J., Sakai, H., Takeuchi, T., and Moriguchi, Y. (1973). Clinical aspect of tardive dyskinesia—especially on the dystonic type. *Ann. Rep. Pharmacother. Res. Found.* 5:205–211.

Klawans, H.L., Jr. (1973a). The pharmacology of extrapyramidal movement disorders. Monograph in Neural Sciences. Vol. 2. S. Karger, Basel.

Klawans, H.L., Jr. (1973b). The pharmacology of tardive dyskinesias. *Am. J. Psychiat.* 130:82-86.

Klawans, H.L., Jr., and Rubovits, R. (1975). The pharmacology of tardive dyskinesia and some animal models, in *Neuropsychopharmacology.* Proceedings of the IX Congress of the Collegium Internationale Neuropsychopharmacologicum, Paris, 7-12 July, 1974. J.R. Boissier, H. Hippius, and R. Pichot, eds. Excerpta Medica American Elsevier Publishing Company, New York. pp. 355-364.

Korsgaard, S. (1976). Baclofen (Lioresal) in the treatment of neuroleptic-induced tardive dyskinesia. *Acta Psychiat. Scand.* 54:17-24.

Lehman, H.F., Ban, T.A., and Saxena, B.M. (1970). A survey of extrapyramidal manifestations in the inpatient population of a psychiatric hospital. *Laval Méd.* 41:909-916.

Moline, R.A. (1975). Atypical tardive dyskinesia. *Am. J. Psychiat.* 132:534-535.

(NIMH) National Institute of Mental Health, Psychopharmacology Research Branch (1975). Development of a dyskinetic movement scale. *ECDEU Intercom.* 4:3-6.

Ogita, K., Yagi, G., Itoh, H., Miura, S., and Lambert, P. (1975). Comparative analysis of persistent dyskinesia of long-term usage with neuroleptics in France and in Japan. *Fol. Psychiat. Neurolog. Jap.* 29:315-320.

Otani, Y., Takase, K., So, Y., et al. (1974). Tardive dyskinesia. *Psychiat. Neurolog. Jap.* 76:310-311.

Parks, J.D. (1976). Clinical aspects of tardive dyskinesia, in *Biochemistry and Neurology.* H.F. Bradford and C.D. Marsden, eds. Academic Press, London. pp. 47-55.

Paulson, G.W. (1968). An evaluation of the permanence of tardive dyskinesia. *Dis. Nerv. Syst.* 29:692-694.

Pryce, I.J., and Edwards, H. (1976). Persistent oral dyskinesia in female mental hospital patients. *Brit. J. Psychiat.* 134:84-87.

Quitkin, F., Rifkin, A., Gochfeld, L., and Klein, F. (1977). Tardive dyskinesia: Are first signs reversible? *Am. J. Psychiat.* 134:84-87.

Rasmussen, S., and Kristensen, M. (1977). Choreoathetosis during phenytoin treatment. *Acta Med. Scand.* 201:239-241.

Roxburgh, P.A. (1977). Treatment of persistent phenothiazine-induced oral dyskinesia. *Brit. J. Psychiat.* 116:277-280.

Sakai, H., Kinoshita, J., and Inose, T. (1972). Tradive dyskinesia: Studies on its clinical survey and postmortem examination of a case. *Ann. Rep. Pharmacopsychiat. Res. Found.* 4:221-229.

Schiele, B.C. (1976). Prevention of tardive dyskinesia. Symposium on Tardive Dyskinesia. Sponsored by Hennepin County Psychiatric Society and Minnesota Psychiatric Society, Minneapolis June 30.

Schönecker, M. (1956). Ein eigentumliches Syndrom im oralen Bereich bei Megaphen Applikation. *Nervenarzt.* 28:35-36.

Seeman, P., Staiman, A., Lee, T., and Chu-Wong, M. (1974). The membrane actions of tranquilizers in relation to neuroleptic-induced parkinsonism and tardive dyskinesia, in The Phenothiazines and Structurally Related Drugs. I.S. Forrest, C.J. Carr, and E. Usdin, eds. Raven Press, New York. pp. 137-148.

Sied, H., and Müller, H.F. (1967). Choreiform movements as side effects of phenothiazine medication in geriatric patients. *J. Am. Geriat. Soc.* 15:517-522.

Sigwald, J., Bouttier, D., Raymondeaud, C., and Piot, C. (1959). Quatre cas de dyskinésie facio-bucco-linguo-masticatrice à évolution prolongée secondaire à un traitment par les neuroléptiques. *Rev. Neurologique.* 10:751-755.

Simpson, G.M., and Kline, N.S. (1976). Tardive dyskinesia: Manifestation, incidence, etiology and treatment, in *The Basal Ganglia*. M.D. Yahr, ed. Raven Press, New York, pp. 427–432.

Simpson, G.M., Lee, J.H., and Shrivastava, R.K. (1978). Clozapine in tardive dyskinesia. *Psychopharmacol.* 56:75–80.

Stafford, J.R., and Fann, W.E. (1977). Deanol acetamidobenzoate (deaner) in tardive dyskinesia. *Dis. Ner. Sys.* 381:12:2:3–6.

Tamminga, C.A., Smith, R.C., Ericksen, S.E., Chang, S., and Davis, J.M. (1977). Cholinergic influences in tardive dyskinesia. *Am. J. Psychiat.* 134:769–774.

Tarsy, D., and Baldessarini, R.J. (1976). The tardive dyskinesia syndrome, in *Clinical Neuropharmacology, Vol. 1.* H.L. Klawans, ed. Raven Press, New York. pp. 29–61.

Tuason, V. (1976). Natural history of tardive dyskinesia. Symposium on Tardive Dyskinesia. Sponsored by Hennepin County Psychiatric Society, Minneapolis, June 30.

Turunen, S. and Achté, K.A. (1967). The bucco-linguo-masticatory syndrome as a side effect of neuroleptics therapy. *Psychiat. Quart.* 41:268–279.

Tzavellas, O., Metzel, E., and Umbach, W. (1967). Uber die Wirksamkeit von α-methyldopa bei Hyperkinesen. *Deutsche Med. Wochen.* 92:1065–1071.

Uhrbrand, L., and Faurbye, A. (1960). Reversible and irreversible dyskinesia after treatment with perphenazine, chlorpromazine, reserpine, and electroconvulsive therapy. *Psychopharmacologia.* 1:408–418.

Villeneuve, A. (1977). Therapeutic trials in tardive dyskinesia. VI World Congress of Psychiatry, Honolulu, Aug. 29.

Villeneuve, A. (1970). The rabbit syndrome. A peculiar extrapyramidal reaction. *Canad. Psychiat. Assn. J.* 17:69–72.

Villenueve, A., and Boszormenyi, A. (1970). Treatment of drug-induced dyskinesias. *Lancet.* Feb. 14:353–354.

Villenueve, A., La Vallee, J.C., and Lemieux, L.H. (1969). Dyskinésie tardive postneuroléptique. *Laval. Med.* 40:832–837.

Wertheimer, J. (1968). Syndrome extrapyramidaux permanents consécutifs à l'administration prolongée de neuroléptiques. *Schweizer Arch. Neurol. Psychiat.* 95:120–173.

Yagi, G., Ogita, K., Ohtsuka, H., Itoh, H., and Miura, S. (1976). Persistent dyskinesia after long-term treatment with neuroleptics in Japan. Its present status and clinical problems. *Keio J. Med.* 25:27–35.

Current Developments in Psychopharmacology, Volume 6
© 1981, Spectrum Publications, Inc.

CHAPTER 5

# NICOTINE AND SMOKING

R. KUMAR
M. LADER

## A. INTRODUCTION

Cigarette smoking is one of the most persistent habits known to man; for many years, he has been possessed by the bizarre but irresistible urge to inhale the smoke produced by burning the dried and shredded leaves of *Nicotiana tabacum*. The alternative methods of administration, sniffing and chewing, lost favor with the introduction of cheap cigarettes made from flue-cured tobacco. Unlike the smoking of cigars and pipes, absorption of nicotine from cigarette smoke mainly takes place in the lungs. Despite convincing evidence that life is shortened by about 5 minutes for every cigarette smoked, consumption continues unabated throughout the world.

If people are asked why they smoke, many reasons are given. In a national survey of adults conducted for the U.S. Public Health Service in 1966, questions were asked about smoking. Six factors were extracted from the data representing the following types of smokers:

1. Habitual—the smoker smokes cigarettes because they are there.
2. Addictive—he smokes to prevent the craving that withdrawal entails.
3. Negative affect reduction—he smokes in order to cope with feelings of anxiety, tension, anger, and aggression in difficult situations.
4. Pleasurable relaxation—to "unwind".
5. Stimulation—to feel energized, alert, and attentive.
6. Sensorimotor manipulation—to have something to do, lighting and handling the cigarette (Ikard et al., 1969).

In a similar English study (McKennell, 1970), a checklist of the main occasions for smoking was administered to smokers and ex-smokers. Factor analysis revealed seven factors. Five were related to within-individual aspects and comprised "nervous irritation," "relaxation," "smoking alone," "activity accompaniment," and "food substitution." Two covered social and social confidence smoking. Russell et al. (1974) mainly confirmed these findings but were unable to find a sedative factor.

Thus, smoking seems to be all things to all smokers. Indeed, it is probable that smokers smoke for different reasons or different combinations of reasons at different times. This raises the crucial issue as to whether these reasons reflect different pharmacological effects of tobacco smoke or whether complex behavioral factors govern smoking behavior. Or, rather, what is the relative contribution of each? The active pharmacological principle in tobacco smoke is nicotine, and it is generally presumed that smokers are seeking the effects of nicotine.

In the following review, such questions are addressed in some detail with reference to:

1. The pharmacology of nicotine in the central nervous system and animal behavior related to these effects.
2. The role of nicotine in smoking behavior in man.
3. The reinforcing properties of nicotine and smoking.

The review is selective both in scope and depth as compendia on the nicotine and smoking literature exist (Larson and Silvette, 1961, 1968, 1971, 1975). The most recent review is that edited by Thornton (1978).*

## B.  STUDIES IN ANIMALS

### 1.  Nicotine Self-Administration

It is estimated that there are some 60 million smokers in the U.S.A. and 20 million in the United Kingdom. Each inhalation of tobacco smoke delivers a bolus of nicotine to the brain within about 7 seconds, and a moderate to heavy smoker probably gives himself over 50,000 such doses of nicotine each year. Despite the immensity of the tobacco smoking habit, there has been a disproportionately small amount of research into the psychopharmacology of smoking and into the role of nicotine. Several recent reviews have pointed to the fact that there is still no conclusive evidence about the very existence of reinforcing actions of nicotine (British Medical Journal, 1977; Kumar and Stolerman, 1977; Jaffe and Jarvik, 1978; Lader, 1978). Some idea of the size of the literature concerned with animal studies of drug self-administration can be obtained by a glance at some recent general reviews of the field (Thompson and Pickens, 1971; Proc. Bayer Symposium, 1973; Proc. Symposium on Control of Drug-Taking Behaviour by Schedules of Reinforcement, 1976; Kumar and Stolerman,

---

*The survey of literature for this review article was concluded on the 1st October 1978.

1977; Martin, 1977a, 1977b; Pickens et al., 1978). The many hundreds of studies of the reinforcing properties of drugs, notably opioids; CNS stimulants, such as the amphetamines and cocaine; sedative/hypnotics, and ethanol stand in stark contrast to the handful of reports of nicotine self-administration. In the case of the hallucinogens, there is also a similar lack of hard evidence of self-administration by animals. However, these drugs are misused relatively rarely and sporadically by man, and it remains to be established whether in their case there results "a state which is characterized by a compulsion to take the drug on a continuous or periodic basis in order to experience its psychic effects, and sometimes to avoid the discomfort of its absence" (Eddy et al., 1964). This type of psychological state is, of course, well known to millions of habitual tobacco smokers, although the evidence for a nicotine abstinence syndrome remains inconclusive (Jaffe and Jarvik, 1978; see also "Nicotine Abstinence Syndrome" later in this chapter).

Deneau and Inoki (1967) reported tests of intravenous self-administration in seven rhesus monkeys, where in most cases it was necessary to "prime" the subjects with repeated programmed injections before they would start responding (pressing a lever) for doses of nicotine (25 $\mu$g/kg nicotine base in saline); a lower dose was not self-administered. The average daily dose that was taken by different monkeys ranged between 0.7 and 1.7 mg/kg nicotine, but individual monkeys showed sharp variations. They often changed their intake by as much as 100 percent on consecutive days, and they tended to take a large dose on one day followed by a small dose the next. In the second phase of the study by these authors, doses were raised at approximately monthly intervals, and although the monkeys responded on the lever less often, their total daily intake nevertheless increased. However, of six survivors, one refused self-administration at the 50 $\mu$g/kg dose level and two stopped at 100 $\mu$g/kg. One monkey each stopped at the 500 $\mu$g/kg and 1000 $\mu$g/kg dose levels, and only one monkey persisted in responding for 2 mg/kg doses; this last animal averaged a daily intake of just under 10 mg/kg and reached a maximum of 14 mg/kg. The maximum rates of responding in this study were seen at the lower doses (up to 68 responses per day); the patterns of responding were variable and the amounts of responding began to decrease as the concentration of nicotine was raised. Perhaps the reductions in response rates were due to the fact that doses of nicotine above 200 $\mu$g/kg produced increasingly severe effects such as yawning, piloerection, flushing and then pallor, mydriasis followed by miosis, dyspnoea, retching, vomiting, and muscular weakness. In the light of such observations, it is surprising that any animals continued to respond. Deneau and Inoki (1967) noted that even at high doses (1.0 and 2.0 mg/kg), these apparently unpleasant effects were very short-lasting, disappearing completely by 20 minutes after the dose. They did not comment on the development of tolerance or lack of it.

There has been one further report of intravenous self-administration of nicotine by monkeys; Yanagita et al. (1974) found that two out of three naive monkeys and all four "self-administration experienced" monkeys initiated and continued intravenous self-administration of nicotine (unit dose 20 μg/kg injection). The monkeys responded only during the "lights on" period (8 A.M. to midnight), and the number of doses taken ranged from an average of 10 a day to 100 a day (i.e., a maximum daily total dose of 2 mg/kg/day). No toxic effects were seen. In another test there was some suggestion that monkeys would respond on a fixed-ratio schedule for large unit doses of nicotine (up to 0.2 mg/kg) but the rates of responding were far less than for cocaine reinforcement. Results of attempts to get monkeys to inhale tobacco smoke were inconclusive.

Clark (1969), in a preliminary report, described oral preferences for nicotine solutions in rats, but the summarized data were of an anecdotal nature. He also reported that 12 rats learned to lever press for intravenous injections of nicotine (10 μg/kg base) after having received repeated pro-grammed injections for a week beforehand. Halving the dose resulted in a 20 percent increase in rate of responding for six rats, but since data for the other six animals were not described, it is not possible to conclude that there was evidence of dose-titration by the rats.

Sanger (1978) substituted solutions of nicotine bitartrate (0.05 mg/ml) for tapwater when measuring schedule-induced polydipsia in four rats. He found that the rats drank less, but nevertheless consumed quite large doses by the oral route, up to 8.5 mg/kg per session. Although the experiment was not primarily concerned with nicotine dependence, it is worth noting that this type of nicotine ingestion does not necessarily reflect nicotine-seeking. A difficulty that is common to all tests of orally ingested doses of nicotine is that a substantial proportion of such doses is metabolized in the first pass through the liver (see also "Effects of Nicotine on Smoking Behavior" following in this chapter).

Recently, Lang et al. (1977) attempted tests in rats of the self-administration of intravenous doses of nicotine and found that the animals would not respond for 0.05 and 0.1 mg/kg doses of nicotine bitartrate. If, however, the rats were food-deprived and then given food pellets at 60-second intervals, i.e., the typical method for schedule-induced polydipsia, they responded more frequently for injections of nicotine than for saline. This interesting observation requires confirmation. It would be important to know what interactions occur between factors such as hunger, the behavi-oral consequences of the food delivery schedule, and the putative reinforcing actions of nicotine. Could such a pattern of responding be blocked by mecamylamine and would the enhanced reinforcing action of nicotine persist in the absence of the food-delivery schedule?

Perhaps in an attempt to answer the criticism that human subjects do not "mainline" nicotine nor drink infusions of this drug, Jarvik (1967) reported some tests of tobacco smoking in monkeys. The animals seemed to puff more frequently at a tube connected to a lit cigarette than at an empty tube, and they preferred cigarette smoke to hot air. There was, however, no evidence to suggest that they inhaled the smoke; the same criticism applies to the study reported by Glick et al. (1970), where four thirsty monkeys were trained to puff at a tube in order to obtain water rewards. Stable rates of puffing were eventually achieved on a fixed-ratio 30 schedule, where two tubes were available: one providing smoke from a permanently available cigarette, and the other providing air. As in Jarvik's experiment (1967), the monkeys preferred the smoke delivery tube. Their rates of puffing and preferences for smoke were then tested after intramuscular injections of mecamylamine, 0.8–3.2 mg/kg. At doses that varied from monkey to monkey, mecamylamine reversed the preferences for smoke without markedly affecting overall rates of puffing, but given the lack of adequate controls, such observations must remain tentative. The interpretation offered was that mecamylamine was blocking the actions of nicotine, which was the rewarding component of the tobacco smoke; thus, only the aversive components of smoke remained. Had there been evidence for actual inhalation of smoke, then, presumably, the putative aversive actions of nicotine would also have been liable to blockade. Such reversals were not confined to mecamylamine, since hexamethonium also produced similar changes. Another puzzling feature of this study was that no increases in smoke preference were seen at low doses of mecamylamine; later tests in human volunteer subjects (Stolerman et al., 1973b) demonstrated increased smoking following medication with mecamylamine.

In summary, the few existing reports of nicotine self-administration by animals are largely of a preliminary nature, and there is little or no systematic evidence about factors that might influence rates of self-administration nor about the ways, if any, in which the drug may be acting as a reinforcer. The remainder of this part of the review will therefore be concerned with behavioral studies in animals which may have some bearing upon questions about possible rewarding actions of nicotine. For example, is nicotine rewarding indirectly because it improves alertness and hence learning and performance, or alternatively, is it reinforcing because it has some sort of tranquilizing action and diminishes responses to stressors? Does nicotine use result in tolerance and abstinence phenomena and might the drug therefore be self-administered to alleviate or avoid abstinence? There seem to be marked individual differences described in studies of motives underlying smoking; are there analogous differences in animals' reactions to doses of nicotine?

## 2. Tests of Spontaneous Motor Activity, Learning, and Performance in Rodents

Nicotine affects the motor activity of rodents in complex ways, and it has not been possible to arrive at descriptive generalizations about the mode of action of this drug in the way that attempts have been made to characterize other drugs, such as amphetamine (Lyon and Robbins, 1975). Nicotine can apparently increase or diminish activity, depending upon interactions between dose and factors such as species (Morrison and Armitage, 1967), strain, and sex (Garg, 1969a; Bättig et al., 1976), or time of day that the tests were done (Bovet-Nitti and Bovet, 1966). Low doses typically increase levels of activity, while higher doses have depressant effects. In general, it seems that animals showing low base-line (undrugged) levels of activity are stimulated by nicotine, while already active animals are either unaffected or are depressed (Morrison and Lee, 1968; Pradhan and Dutta, 1970), but there are some contradictory findings (Garg, 1969a). Attempts have been made to link the stimulant or depressant effects of nicotine with actions on forebrain serotonin metabolism in rats showing high or low base-line levels of activity (Rosecrans, 1971). But since nicotine almost certainly exerts equally important effects on dopamine and nor-adrenaline as well as on acetylcholine, one is obliged, in the present state of knowledge, to agree with Jaffe and Jarvik (1978) that "effects on neurotransmitters do not provide significant insights into the ways in which nicotine reinforces smoking behaviour." Similarly, there is a temptation to draw parallels between the subtle and variable ways in which nicotine can modify learned and unlearned responses in animals and the variety of reasons that smokers give for smoking. Human typologies of smoking behavior (Tomkins, 1966; Ikard et al., 1969; Russell et al., 1974) characterize smokers in a number of overlapping ways (see also "Introduction"), but some other independent characteristics, e.g. of a physiological nature, or in terms of responses to drugs other than nicotine, should also be shown to co-vary with the different motivational types of "smoking personalities" that are derived from such studies.

In a test of bar-pressing by rats for water rewards, Morrison et al. (1969) found that, typically, injections of nicotine (0.4 mg/kg of the base) initially depressed responding, and that about 30 minutes later there was a facilitation of the rate of bar-pressing. Mecamylamine blocked both effects of nicotine, whereas atropine antagonized only the initial depressant action. It seemed therefore that in addition to producing muscarinic actions of acetylcholine, nicotine was also either stimulating (unidentified) nicotinic receptors, or perhaps acting indirectly through some other mechanisms such as release of catecholamines. These possibilities were, however, not examined directly. In a similar study, Domino and Lutz (1973) have shown that tolerance develops rapidly to the initial suppressant actions of nicotine on responding by rats for water rewards. Although these workers did not demonstrate subsequent facilitation of behavior, it would be interesting to compare the reactions of nicotine naive and tolerant rats on such tests when given drugs such as mecamylamine and atropine, and substances affecting other neurotransmitters.

In addition to differences in responsiveness related to time since medication (Morrison et al., 1969), other observations on the effects of nicotine on learned behavior are also broadly consistent with tests of spontaneous activity, in that the drug tends to increase low base-line rates of responding (Morrison, 1967, 1968; Pradhan and Dutta, 1970); while high rates are either unaffected (Morrison, 1967) or reduced (Stitzer et al., 1970). Similarly, the acquisition of some behavioral responses, e.g., shuttle-box avoidance, is also facilitated in strains of animals that are normally "poor" avoiders (Bovet et al., 1966, 1967). In tests of the performance of pole-jump avoidance, Domino (1973) noted that with subcutaneous doses of nicotine base above 0.25 mg/kg, there were consistent and selective depressions of avoidance, while escape behavior remained relatively unaffected. Such a differential effect was reminiscent of the profile of actions obtained with chlorpromazine, morphine, and tetrahydrocannabinol. While recognizing that there was a hundredfold or more differences between the amounts of nicotine given by injection and those obtained by inhaling smoke, Domino (1973) wondered whether nicotine might not also have some "tranquilizing" actions. The empirical nature of the pole-jump test and the varied actions of the reference drugs notwithstanding, this is an interesting speculation which is taken up in more detail elsewhere in this review ("Nicotine Reinforcement and Arousal").

An alternative possibility is that nicotine is a "stimulant" rather than a tranquilizer, and in an experiment aimed at mimicking the sort of dose that is normally inhaled by taking a puff (equivalent to 1–2 $\mu$g/kg nicotine base given intravenously), Armitage et al. (1968) showed that intermittent, small, intravenous doses of nicotine usually increased rates of bar-pressing by thirsty rats for water rewards. The speed of injection and the interval between injections were critical factors, but it was felt that under selected conditions of dose and timing, these "smoking doses" of nicotine were producing some kind of central stimulant effects which, in turn, were responsible for the elevated rates of responding. Such an effect on performance might have some relevance to the facilitations of learning seen both in tests of avoidance behavior (Bovet et al., 1966, 1967) or following post-trial injections of nicotine in maze-learning tasks (Garg, 1969b). Repeated intravenous injections of "smoking doses" of nicotine in anesthetized cats resulted both in electrocortical desynchronization and in an increase in the release of acetylcholine from the cortex (Armitage et al., 1968). It was suggested, therefore, that inhaled nicotine might be reinforcing because of its alerting actions. Such actions would depend critically upon the baseline, i.e., concentration and efficiency might only improve if they were previously low. On the other hand, a smoker who was overaroused might seek a depressant effect of nicotine, e.g., by increasing the dose inhaled. Armitage et al. (1968) commented that "someone smoking a cigarette has literally finger-tip control of how much nicotine he takes into his mouth; by reducing the puff volume, or inhaling less frequently, he absorbs less nicotine." At first sight, such an hypothesis seems very attractive; nicotine is a drug that has both depressant and stimulant effects on behavior and on cortical activation, effects that depend critically upon dose and time. Since an individual's arousal level and efficiency are likely to fluctuate spontaneously as well as in response to environmental events, nicotine can be regarded as an all-purpose modulator, by the use of which a smoker keeps his requirements for stimulation and sedation constantly tuned to perfection. It is, however, virtually impossible to prove or disprove such an all-embracing hypothesis, which can easily adapt post-hoc to accommodate almost any new data, particularly if they do not extend to more than three or four points on a hypothetical inverted-U continuum.

## 3.   Nicotine, Reinforcement, and "Arousal"

There are several animal studies that bear directly on the question of arousal and nicotine reinforcement. Bradley and Elkes (1957) recorded electrical activity from different brain regions of various experimental preparations of cats and monkeys, e.g., conscious, encephale isolé, cerveau isolé, anesthetized. They concluded that while cholinergic neurones were present throughout the brainstem activating system, nicotinic neurones were to be found only in the mid-brain reticular formation. Yamamoto and Domino (1965) tested the effects of intravenous nicotine in cats with chronically implanted electrodes in the amygdala, hippocampus, posterior hypothalamus, mesencephalic reticular formation, and on the surface of the somatosensory cortex. They compared the (+) and (−) isomers of nicotine and found that the (+) isomer was ineffective. The (−) isomer, on the other hand, produced both behavioral and electroencephalographic (EEG) arousal, followed a few minutes later by slow wave sleep. The first EEG sign of arousal was the emergence of hippocampal theta rhythm, and this arousal-inducing action of nicotine was blocked by mecamylamine. Domino (1967), using mid-, or high-pontine preparations in several species, found that doses of nicotine, ranging from 5–20 $\mu$g/kg intravenously, resulted in EEG activation. In line with other speculations, e.g., by Armitage et al. (1968), he wondered whether these arousing effects were in any way relevant to the facilitations of learning seen in the acquisition of pole-jump avoidance by "slow" rats.

Armitage and Hall (1968) calculated that when a smoker inhaled a puff, he was probably taking the equivalent of an intravenous dose on the order of 1-2 $\mu$g/kg. These workers then delivered puffs of smoke, which approximately mimicked human puffed doses, into the tracheas of encephale isolé cats. After about eight such puffs they observed signs of behavioral arousal, e.g., opening of eyes, reactions to visual stimuli, movements of ears and vibrissae, and, at the same time, desynchronization of cortical activity.

Routtenberg (1968) proposed a "two-arousal" hypothesis in which the reticular formation and the limbic system were seen as functioning in a mutually inhibitory manner. The reticular formation was believed to be mediating non-specific or generalized arousal, whereas the limbic structures were involved in the activation of goal-directed, incentive-oriented behaviors. Nelsen and her colleagues have reported a series of studies in which they link the effects of repeated medication with nicotine, both with improvements in goal-directed responding (Nelsen and Goldstein, 1972) and with increasing dominance of the hypothesized limbic arousal mechanisms. A shift, it was argued, in the control of cortical arousal from the reticular formation to the hippocampus in rabbits (Bhattacharya and Goldstein, 1970), was consistent with behavioral observations in rats in that the subjects, when injected repeatedly with nicotine, 100 $\mu$g/kg subcutaneously, made fewer inappropriate responses on a lever-pressing task. In a later study, Nelsen et al. (1975) reported that electrical stimulation of the reticular formation, via chronically implanted electrodes, disrupted performance of a lever-pressing task involving visual "attention" in rats. This effect was attenuated by acute subcutaneous medication with nicotine base, 100 $\mu$g/kg. The results of such experiments have not yet been confirmed, and more detailed studies of chronic medication with nicotine are needed to test and refine hypotheses linking nicotine with arousal, incentive, and performance. It is suggested, for example, that some smokers may not be inhaling to arouse or alert themselves (see Domino, 1967; Armitage and Hall, 1968); but rather that by activating another brain system, they damp down reticular-activating mechanisms. In this context, Friedman et al. (1974) have suggested that smokers lower their arousal level by attenuating sensory input; but fuller comparisons are needed in man with intravenous or aerosol doses of nicotine, which are obtained independently of smoking behavior, before such interpretations are fully acceptable.

An extension of the arousal-reduction hypotheses was put forward by Hall and Morrison (1973); these workers reported tests in which rats pressed levers in order to avoid electric shocks. Rats were trained, either drugged with nicotine or with saline. Both groups learned the response, and there was some early facilitation of responding by nicotine. However, when saline was substituted for the nicotine, there were disruptions in performance, and it was suggested that nicotine might be maintaining successful levels of performance because it diminished the subjects' responses to stress. In support of the stress-relief hypothesis, it was argued that since intravenous or intraventricular nicotine caused a release of noradrenaline from the hypothalamus (Hall and Turner, 1972), this in turn might inhibit the release of corticosteroids from the adrenal cortex (Van Loon et al., 1971). Subsequent reports (Balfour et al., 1975) have not supported the suggestion that nicotine might reduce corticosteroid secretion in stressed rats. Some further behavioral tests (Balfour and Morrison, 1975) have indicated that nicotine both facilitates avoidance responding and increases adrenal weight in rats. It is therefore not yet clear how nicotine acts on the pituitary-adrenal system in stressed or unstressed subjects. There are as yet no experimental findings to support the hypothesis that nicotine is self-administered in order to diminish responses to stressors.

## 4.  Nicotine and Brain Mechanisms of Reward

The amine-releasing properties of nicotine are not well understood. Studies in animals indicate that nicotine can cause changes in turnover and release of both dopamine and noradrenaline from the brain (Sulser and Sanders-Bush, 1971; Goodman, 1974; Westfall, 1974; Giorguieff et al., 1976; Lichtensteiger et al., 1976; De Belleroche and Bradford, 1978); and in addition to markedly altering the cortical release of acetylcholine (Armitage et al., 1969), nicotine also affects the turnover of serotonin (Rosecrans, 1971) as well as the uptake and release of both serotonin and noradrenaline by the hippocampus and hypothalamus (Balfour, 1973). The functional significance of such effects, in terms of consummatory responding (see Münster and Bättig, 1975) remains virtually unexplored, and there have been very few studies of the effects of nicotine on intracranial self-stimulation behavior (ICSS). It is well known that rats with electrodes placed either in the lateral or the posterior hypothalamus will respond to electrical stimulation, and it has been shown that nicotine can facilitate ICSS (Wanner and Bättig, 1966; Olds and Domino, 1969; Pradhan and Bowling, 1971; Newman, 1972). Consistent with observations on responding for other types of reinforcers (see review by Sanger and Blackman, 1976), Pradhan and Bowling (1971) also found rate-dependent effects with ICSS; the lower the response rate, the more pronounced was the facilitating effect of nicotine. In rats that had high base-line rates of responding, it was found that nicotine could still exert facilitating effects if the rate was artificially lowered by reducing the intensity of the reinforcing current. The facilitation by nicotine was blocked by mecamylamine and also by pretreatment with reserpine. It was therefore concluded (Pradhan and Bowling, 1971; German and Bowden, 1974) that nicotine was probably mediating its facilitatory effect on ICSS through the release of noradrenaline, although other interpretations are possible for the effects of reserpine pretreatment. Newman (1972) concurred with the idea that nicotine facilitated ICSS through actions on an activating noradrenergic "go" system, and that the other part of the cholinergic influence on ICSS was a reciprocal, inhibitory "no-go" component, which was muscarinic in nature. Dose-dependent facilitating effects of nicotine were, however, not demonstrable as was the case with drugs such as amphetamine (Domino and Olds, 1972). There do not seem to have been further investigations of nicotine and ICSS, and this apparent lack of interest is surprising in the light of recent general developments in this field relating to more specific identification of anatomical and chemical substrates of brain reward as well as refinements of hypotheses about incentive and reinforcement mechanisms (German and Bowden, 1974; Crow and Deakin, 1978; Wise, 1978).

## 5.  Comments on Studies of Site of Action of Nicotine in the CNS

Although there is general agreement that Renshaw cells in the spinal cord possess nicotinic receptors, very little is known about the presence and distribution of similar receptor sites elsewhere in the central nervous system. Recent binding studies using constituents of certain snake neurotoxins, e.g., α-bungarotoxin (α-BT) and Naja naja toxin, have raised the possibility that sites analogous to peripheral nicotinic acetylcholine receptors can be mapped in the brain (Salvaterra et al., 1975; Speth et al., 1977; Morley et al., 1977; Moore and Brady, 1977; Hunt and Schmidt, 1978; Schechter et al., 1978). There are, however, some findings that suggest that central nicotinic receptors and toxin-binding molecules may not be one and the same. For example, studies of [14]C-labeled nicotine accumulation in brain slice preparations (Goodman, 1974; Weiss and Alderdice, 1975; Alderdice and Weiss, 1975) suggest that there is some specific mechanism for sequestering nicotine, and that mecamylamine competes with nicotine. However, the binding of α-BT to brain sites, although diminished by acetylcholine, nicotine, curare, and decamethonium, was not affected by atropine or mecamylamine (Morley et al., 1977). Furthermore, α-BT was found not to block the responses of Renshaw cells to acetylcholine (Duggan et al., 1976), and there was a similar lack of effect on sympathetic ganglia (Brown and Fumagalli, 1977). On the other hand, there is some anatomical correlation between brain regions, which show the presence or absence of toxin-binding, and the occurrence or lack of "nicotinic" activity, e.g., the hippocampus and the caudate nucleus, respectively (Schechter et al., 1978). Tests of stereospecific binding of nicotine itself (Martin et al., 1978) may help to clarify the nature and distribution of putative nicotinic receptors in the brain, and thus lead to improved methods for studying the behavioral actions of nicotine.

## 6.  Nicotine as a Discriminative Stimulus

Morrison and Stephenson (1969) trained rats to make a saline-nicotine discrimination, and then showed it could be blocked by a central antagonist (chlorisondamine). Very similar findings were later reported by Schechter and Rosecrans (1971), using a T-maze procedure. The nicotine cue waned over time after injection, and it was found that 60 minutes after dosing, rats which had learned to respond correctly shortly after injections of nicotine or saline now responded randomly (Schechter and Jellinek, 1975). In a series of studies using a two-lever operant task—similar to that described by Morrison and Stephenson (1969)—Rosecrans and his colleagues have presented strong evidence that nicotine can assume stimulus control of operant behavior: When drugged with nicotine the rats learn to respond on one lever only, and when given saline they respond on the other (Hirschhorn and Rosecrans, 1974). The nicotine cue was blocked in such tests by mecamylamine; other tests of the antagonism of the central nicotine cue showed that of a range of other possible antagonists or drugs that interfered with neurotransmitter functioning—hexamethonium, atropine, dibenamine, propranolol, α-methyl-paratyrosine, and p-chlorophenylalanine—only α-methyl-paratyrosine had some blocking effect in one study but not in another. Such an action might well have reflected a more generalized effect, and Rosecrans and Chance (1977) concluded that nicotine was acting on some specific cholinergic receptors independent of catechol and indoleamine systems. Other tests also summarized by Rosecrans and Chance (1977) have aimed to use more specific measures to deplete brain noradrenaline and dopamine. The effects of noradrenaline depletion in some ways suggested an increased sensitivity to nicotine, while rats deficient in dopamine showed some impairments in their ability to respond to the nicotine cue.

### 7. Studies of Tolerance to Nicotine

Morrison and Stephenson (1972) measured the locomotor activity of rats by an automated method and found that nicotine had an initial depressant effect followed by an increase above control levels. As the experiment progressed, it was found, following repeated medication, that the initial depression of activity became less and less apparent and, eventually, the action of nicotine became predominantly stimulant. Controls were incorporated for the effects of habituation to the apparatus. When animals were retested after an interval of 23 days, there was still some evident tolerance to nicotine. Keenan and Johnson (1972) also tested the effects of repeated doses of nicotine on motor activity, and their results were broadly consistent with those of Morrison and Stephenson (1972); in addition, on cessation of nicotine treatment, they described a "rebound" increase in the amounts of rearing.

In a study of locomotor activity in rats Stolerman et al. (1973a) showed that ambulation and rearing were reduced in a dose-related way. When rats were injected repeatedly for 3 days and then "challenged" with nicotine, the depressant action was greatly reduced. There were no signs of abstinence in nicotine pretreated rats, which were then tested with saline. Hatchell and Collins (1977) have subsequently demonstrated in mice that subjects' sex and strain can influence the development of tolerance. In the tests by Stolerman et al. (1973a), it was also found that there was persisting evidence of tolerance 80 days after the end of the nicotine treatment. In a later experiment, Stolerman et al. (1974) showed that tolerance could be demonstrated even if repeated injections of nicotine was spaced widely apart, in this case at intervals of 3 days. The prolonged changes after repeated medication might be consistent with persistently altered metabolic responses, which have been reported in human ex-smokers (Beckett and Triggs, 1967). Rosenthal and Slotkin (1977) have shown that a very large single dose of nicotine given to neonatal rats produces changes in catecholamine biosynthesis for up to 23 days. Studies in animals of the effects of chronic medication with nicotine (Bhagat, 1970a,b; Bhagat et al., 1971) have shown some gross changes, such as increased adrenal weights, and there are also indications of an increased turnover of brain noradrenaline; Westfall et al. (1967) have reported variable changes in brain levels of serotonin.

Tests of learned behavior have also been used to demonstrate the development of tolerance to the depressant effects of nicotine. Domino and Lutz (1973) found that a dose of 0.25 mg/kg nicotine base initially suppressed bar-pressing by rats for water rewards. With repeated daily tests, the rats began pressing after shorter and shorter delays following their injections, but at no stage was there any facilitation of responding. There is no evidence for or against the notion that changes in such "depressant" actions of nicotine may parallel the development of tolerance to the adverse effects of the drug in man, especially nausea (Johnston, 1942; Rottenstein et al., 1960; Beckett et al., 1971). There has been very little systematic research into the aversive properties of nicotine, in spite of the fact that it is widely held that tolerance to such effects is a necessary step before smokers can go on to inhale increasing amounts of nicotine in the process of becoming dependent (see Russell, 1977).

Nelsen and Goldstein (1972) tested rats on an "attention" task, based upon the procedure described by Kornetsky and Eliasson (1969) in which two types of error are recorded: those of omission and of commission. This is a difficult test in which animals must not only respond correctly in the presence of a given stimulus, but they must also withold responses at other times. Acute doses of nicotine (100 $\mu$g/kg base) impaired performance generally, but repeated testing against a background of chronic medication showed that while there were no systematic changes due to nicotine treatment on omission errors, errors of commission decreased and there was even a suggestion of improvement above base-line levels. The authors commented that "chronic nicotine treatment improved the efficiency of response to goal-oriented or incentive-oriented stimuli without causing or being accompanied by a generalized increase in the level of activity." This particular study is important because it attempts to examine the effects of chronic nicotine treatment in relation to mechanisms of attention and arousal, although the findings have not yet been confirmed or extended.

Tolerance may develop at different rates to different actions of nicotine, and experiments in rats suggest that tolerance to the effects of nicotine can be detected as a central cue. Schechter and Rosecrans (1972), using a T-maze task, found that repeated, frequent injections of nicotine markedly impaired the ability of rats to make correct responses, depending on whether they had just been given an injection of nicotine or saline.

*"Acute" Tolerance to Nicotine*

Aside from possible metabolic disturbances after repeated or very large single doses of nicotine, some other physiological changes may underly the altered sensitivity to nicotine after single, relatively small doses. Stolerman et al. (1973a) have shown a reduction in sensitivity to the locomotor depressant actions of "challenge" doses of nicotine, which reaches a peak up to 2 hours after pretreatment and then wanes over the next 6 hours. The time course of acute tolerance on such behavioral tests cannot easily be reconciled with earlier observations by Domino (1967), who found that if intravenous doses of nicotine were spaced apart at intervals of greater than 30 minutes, then tolerance to the EEG-activating effects of nicotine could not be detected. However, in a more recent study (Hubbard and Gohd, 1975), there was evidence of tolerance on measures of behavioral and EEG arousal after small doses of nicotine spaced one day apart. Very little seems to be known about the physiological changes that may underlie acute and prolonged tolerance after single or repeated doses of nicotine.

## 8. Nicotine Abstinence Syndrome

The phenomena of tolerance and abstinence generally go hand in hand and form the basis for understanding some aspects of drug dependence (see review by Kumar and Stolerman, 1977). In their recent review, Jaffe and Jarvik (1978) observe that "a variety of psychological, behavioral, and physiological disturbances have been reported to follow the discontinuation of smoking. Among the symptoms reported following the cessation of smoking, in addition to the craving for tobacco, are irritability, restlessness, dullness, sleep disturbances, gastrointestinal disturbances, drowsiness, headache, amnesia, anxiety; and impairment of concentration, judgement, and psychomotor performance. The onset of such symptoms usually occurs within a matter of hours or days after smoking cessation, and have been reported to last from days to months. In spite of this impressive collection of symptoms and a variety of signs, such as changes in EEG (Ulett and Itil, 1969; Vasquez and Toman, 1967), muscle tension (Hutchinson and Emley, 1973), and weight gain (W.H.O., 1975), reliable animal models of the nicotine abstinence syndrome are conspicuous by their absence. Jaffe and Jarvik (1978) cite two studies in animals, in one of which (Seevers, 1973), no significant signs of withdrawal were seen following abrupt cessation of nicotine medication in monkeys. Hutchinson and Emley (1973), however, found that monkeys became more irritable on being withdrawn from nicotine.

Larson and Silvette (1975), in their comprehensive review, cite Bernstein (1970) who commented, "There was no evidence from human studies to support the notion that a consistent, characteristic withdrawal syndrome occurs in all or even most individuals who discontinue smoking." And they then add, "Had we the technique to measure the response of a neuron deprived of its once-nicotine-containing milieu, we would possess visible evidence as striking as the convulsions which are part of the barbiturate abstinence syndrome." The paradox is that behavioral and physiological techniques that are highly sensitive in the case of other drugs *are* available, and still the putative nicotine abstinence syndrome continues to elude definition and description.

## C. STUDIES IN HUMANS

### 1. Measurement of Nicotine and Carboxyhaemoglobin Concentrations

#### a. Nicotine

The study of nicotine and smoking behavior in humans was long hampered by the inability to measure nicotine concentrations in biological fluids. Consequently, the pharmacokinetic, and to some extent the pharmacodynamic, aspects of nicotine actions in man were poorly understood. The development of gas chromatographic techniques for estimating nicotine (McNiven et al., 1965; Beckett and Triggs, 1966) has helped elucidate the role of nicotine in smoking. Using such a technique with a flame-ionization detector, Isaac and Rand (1972) attained a sensitivity of 1 ng/ml of nicotine in a 2.5 ml sample. In six male habitual smokers, plasma-nicotine concentrations averaged 2.7 ng/ml before smoking (range 1–8) and 20.7 ng/ml (range 12–44) 30 minutes after smoking the last cigarette in a 6.5 hour ad libitum smoking session. Next, subjects refrained from smoking for 8 hours and then smoked one of their preferred brands of cigarettes at the rate of one puff a minute. The amount of nicotine extracted from the smoke was calculated from the difference between the nicotine contents of exhaled and inhaled smoke and ranged from 0.86 to 3.12 mg. The maximal level to which the plasma nicotine rose was related to the amount of nicotine extracted ($r = 0.88$; $p <0.02$). However, the amount extracted could differ greatly from the estimated nicotine yield of the cigarette, as measured with a standard smoking machine. This illustrates the crude nature of nicotine yield as a relevant parameter in smoking experiments. Butt length and nicotine content are also only crude ways of estimating nicotine intake in a smoker.

The plasma half-life of nicotine was less than 30 minutes, but cumulation quickly occurred in smokers smoking a cigarette every 30 minutes (Armitage, 1978). In spite of this, the rate of elimination is high enough for nicotine levels to drop substantially overnight, so that day-to-day accumulation does not occur.

Russell's group has introduced almost routine monitoring of plasma-nicotine concentrations in their various studies manipulating smoking behavior (Feyerabend et al., 1975). They confirmed that smoking a single cigarette produces a rise in plasma-nicotine concentration of about 25 ng/ml. Peak levels were higher in men (38 ng/ml) than in women (27 ng/ml) (Russell et al., 1976a).

In another study (Russell et al., 1975b) 10 regular cigarette smokers continued to smoke their usual brand (mean yield 1.34 mg nicotine), or were switched to high-yield (3.2 mg) or low-yield (0.14 mg) cigarettes each for a day. The plasma-nicotine level 2 minutes after a normal cigarette in the mid-morning (before any switch) was 24.4 ng/ml with a range of 15.5–38.4 ng/ml among the smokers. Variation between days for each smoker was much less. There was no relation between the mid-morning nicotine level and the subjects' usual cigarette consumption or the nicotine yield of their usual brand of cigarette. When changed to a low-nicotine cigarette for a day, consumption rose only slightly. However, significantly fewer high-yield cigarettes were smoked on the test day (a fall from 10.8 to 6.7 per day). Average afternoon levels of nicotine were no different from morning levels for normal cigarettes (30.1 as compared with 24.4 ng/ml in the morning) or high-yield ones (29.2 as compared with 24.4 ng/ml). After switching to low-nicotine cigarettes, levels dropped to 8.5 ng/ml. Variation was great, especially after switching to high-yield cigarettes, but it seemed that the adjustment was more in terms of the way the cigarette was smoked than the number, as the nicotine levels and number of cigarettes smoked stayed roughly the same. Again the nicotine yield of the cigarette as gauged from standard smoking machines was a misleading indication of potential smoking behavior, showing no correlation to plasma-nicotine peaks.

More recently, Russell and Feyerabend (1978) have reported on plasma-nicotine concentrations during prolonged heavy smoking—three 1.3 mg nicotine cigarettes per hour for 7 hours. Concentrations rose over the first 3 hours, but then reached a steady-state around 40–50 ng/ml. Even so, peaks and troughs associated with each cigarette were still identifiable. In another part of this study, plasma concentrations after repeated intravenous injections of nicotine were estimated. Nicotine peaks did not alter with repeated injections, yet the concomitant tachycardias fell off markedly, suggesting a tachyphylactic effect.

## b. Carboxyhaemoglobin Concentrations

Another blood estimation that has proved of value is the carboxyhaemoglobin level (COHb). The COHb level rose with every cigarette smoked by about 1.3 per cent and fell between cigarettes, but remained fairly constant otherwise throughout the day (Castleden and Cole, 1974). Therefore, a random COHb estimation was a fairly good indicator of the mean level of smoking maintained by a subject. One precaution is that an estimate should not be taken within 30 minutes of smoking a cigarette, as it takes this time for the carbon monoxide to attain distribution equilibrium in the extravascular compartments of the body. COHb levels are consistently higher in smokers than non-smokers, even during the night, and are a fair reflection of the amount of cigarette smoke inhaled over an integral period of time.

Russell et al. (1973b), in their study of subjects switching to high and low nicotine-yield cigarettes, found that COHb levels fell in both cases. The decrease on switching to high-yield cigarettes was attributed to the drop in the number of cigarettes smoked, the CO yield per cigarette remaining roughly the same. With the low-yield cigarettes, the CO delivery per cigarette was much lower also, which accounted for the drop in COHb levels.

Manufactured cigarettes vary greatly in their CO yield (Russell et al., 1975a). For example, the mean increase after smoking a single cigarette was 1.45 per cent for a standard-size brand (10 puffs) and 1.09 per cent for a small-size brand (7 puffs). For extra-mild cigarettes, the increases were 0.64 and 0.75 per cent, respectively, much more than the proportionate nicotine decrease (1.2 and 0.3 mg nicotine per cigarette) (Russell et al., 1973a). Data such as these have led to demands that the CO yield of available brands of cigarettes be published as well as tar and nicotine yields. However, CO yields themselves depend on the puffing pattern, and this varies greatly from individual to individual and with different types of cigarettes. Puffing rate is highest at the beginning of a cigarette and then slows down, possibly because the nicotine and tar in the stub become more concentrated as the cigarette burns down. This is reflected in a rapid rise of COHb concentrations at the start of a cigarette followed by a leveling off or even a fall toward the end of the cigarette (Ashton and Telford, 1973).

Despite these problems, COHb blood-concentration estimations provide a useful check on manipulations designed to reduce cigarette smoking in real-life conditions. With nicotine chewing gums, for example, COHb levels dropped less than expected as recorded cigarette consumption fell off (Table 3), suggesting a change in pattern of inhalation (Russell et al., 1976b).

## 2. Effect of Nicotine on Smoking Behavior

### a. By Injection

In the earliest of these few studies, Johnston (1942) gave nicotine injections hypodermically to 35 volunteers. Some received single doses, but most had multiple doses. After 1.3 mg of nicotine, non-smokers termed the effects "queer," with muzziness and light-headedness being commonly reported. Smokers, however, "invariably thought the sensation pleasant and, given an adequate dose, were disinclined for a smoke for some time thereafter." A dose of 1.6 mg usually produced toxic symptoms in non-smokers, whereas heavy inhalers or pipe smokers easily tolerated 6.5 mg injections. Intravenous injections of 0.14 to 0.21 mg of nicotine (possibly as the tartrate) closely simulated the subjective effects of a deep inhalation. The nicotine action was perceived in about 15 sec., both on inhalation of tobacco smoke and on intravenous injection of nicotine and lasted for 1 or 2 minutes. Johnston gave himself 3 to 4 daily subcutaneous injections of 1.3 mg of nicotine for 20 days and found himself preferring these to smoking.

A study frequently cited as proving the crucial role of nicotine in smoking behavior is that of Lucchesi et al. (1967). Subjects received nicotine via a slow intravenous infusion, but were unaware of the nature of the drug. They were allowed to smoke, the number and the butt weight of the cigarettes being measured. In the first experiment, 4 subjects received 1 mg of nicotine bitartrate over 20 minutes: smoking behavior was not affected. Next, 5 subjects were given 2 mg of nicotine bitartrate in the first hour and 4 mg during each of the next 5 hours (totaling 22 mg over 6 hours, which is equivalent to about 7 mg of nicotine base). There was a 27 per cent reduction in the number of cigarettes smoked, compared with saline infusion—from 10 to 7.3 cigarettes over the 6 hours (p < 0.001). Butt weights increased 20 per cent and the subjects took fewer puffs. Finally, 4 subjects received 8 mg of nicotine bitartrate over 6 hours, which increased heart rate but did not alter smoking behavior. Thus, infusion rates of 4 mg per hour or so were needed to reduce smoking. The authors comment, "We should have observed a much greater reduction in the smoking frequency." But the infusion rate was only equivalent to about 1 to 2 cigarettes per hour, and marked suppression was thus unlikely.

However, slow infusion does not mimic the repeated bolus effects that successive puffs and inhalations produce. In an attempt to simulate cigarette smoking more closely, we gave the nicotine in 10 bolus injections (Kumar et al., 1977). First, we established that "forced puffing" on a high or an average nicotine content cigarette, as compared with puffing on a nicotine-free herbal cigarette, produced a dose-related diminution in the number of puffs on a freely available lighted cigarette during the subsequent 10 minutes (Table 1). The volume per puff was also diminished, and physiological effects were detected in the form of heart-rate increases and augmentation of the fast-wave (beta) activity in the EEG. In the second part of the experiment, nicotine bitartrate or saline was injected as 10 boluses to a total of 1.7 mg, 0.85 mg, and 0 mg/70 kg body weight of nicotine base over 10 minutes. Again, tachycardia and increase in EEG beta were produced in a dose-related manner. Surprisingly, no effect on the smoking behavior was produced. This unexpected result suggests that, under the conditions of our experiment, nicotine was not the sole, nor even the main, reinforcer of smoking. This study is being repeated with estimations of plasma nicotine as an additional and important measure.

### b. By Inhalation

The most appropriate way to attempt to mimic the inhalation characteristics of the cigarette smoker is to administer nicotine by aerosol. There are problems in aerosol particle size, pH of the solution, rate of delivery, and acceptability to the subject. That the approach is feasible is shown by a study in which two puffs from a nicotine aerosol (1.06 mg) seemed to compare with a single inhalation from a lighted cigarette (Herxheimer, Griffiths, Hamilton and Wakefield, 1967). In fact, similar increases in pulse rate and blood pressure were obtained in each instance. The mean pulse rate increase with the cigarette was 9.8 beats/min, with the aerosol 8.0; the corresponding figures for systolic and diastolic blood pressure were 5.2/3.2 and 6.7/7.9. The effects became apparent 1 or 2 minutes after the subject started to inhale nicotine, but the peak effect was earlier with the aerosol. No systematic

**Table 1. Effects of Nicotine Given by Inhalation and by Bolus Injections, as Compared with Placebo, on Smoking Behavior and Physiological Activity\*†**

| | | Mode of Administration | | | | | |
|---|---|---|---|---|---|---|---|
| | | Inhalation | | | Injection | | |
| Variable | Dose Level: | 0 | Low | High | 0 | Low | High |
| Number of puffs/10 min | | 8.00 | 6.70 | 4.80 | 10.00 | 8.80 | 9.50 |
| Volume/puff (ml) | | 36.00 | 29.00 | 26.00 | 16.00 | 17.00 | 16.00 |
| Heart rate/min | | 75.90 | 77.20 | 79.30 | 73.50 | 76.00 | 78.20 |
| Beta voltage ($\mu$V) | | 1.92 | 1.94 | 2.07 | 1.57 | 1.70 | 1.80 |

\* Abstracted from Kumar et al. (1977).
† Nicotine was administered at 2 dose levels, and effects were noted during the ensuing 10 minutes.

studies of aerosol nicotine effects on smoking behavior have been reported.

### c. By Mouth

This route of administration is ambiguously termed because it can refer to oral ingestion with absorption in the gastrointestinal tract or to buccal absorption, the drug being retained in the mouth. Nicotine tartrate (10 mg) in capsules or placebo capsules was administered 5 times a day on alternate days. On any given day, all five capsules were either nicotine or placebo. The average number of cigarettes dropped marginally but significantly from a mean of 24.1 on placebo days to 22.4 on nicotine days. However, the average butt weight per cigarette and ratings of strength and quality of the cigarettes were not altered (Jarvik et al., 1970). Although the authors interpret the weak effect as pointing to the "important role played by secondary conditioning," there is no evidence that the nicotine was actually absorbed, or if absorbed, that it was not extensively metabolized first-pass before reaching the systemic circulation.

Buccal absorption has the advantage of avoiding such metabolism, and nicotine-containing chewing gums have been formulated (Fernö et al., 1973), but proved disappointing in clinical trials as a smoking substitute (Brant-mark et al., 1973). Using a similar preparation, Jarvik's group administered placebo gum, or low-yield (1 mg) or high-yield (4 mg) nicotine gum to 56 undergraduate subjects and compared the effects on latency to lighting up the next cigarette and puff times with those of nil, low- (0.3 mg), and high-nicotine (1.3 mg) content cigarettes (Kozlowski et al., 1975). The subjects were unaware that the experiment concerned smoking behavior. The latency to lighting up the next standard cigarette was less after smoking low- rather than high-nicotine content cigarettes, but was not affected by gum nicotine content (Table 2). Conversely, the puff times were unaffected by prior smoking of test cigarettes, but were curtailed when a high-nicotine gum had been chewed (Table 2).

There were complications in the design and execution of this experiment, which render its interpretation difficult, but the authors ventured the opinion that pharmacokinetic differences in buccal and alveolar absorption were responsible for the differential effects on latency and puff times. The lack of plasma-nicotine levels is particularly unfortunate here.

Nicotine gum has also been evaluated as an aid to giving up smoking, but with pharmacokinetic controls sufficient to provide information about the role of nicotine in smoking behavior (Russell et al., 1976b). Forty-three smokers wishing to give up smoking were administered nicotine-containing gum (2 mg) or placebo gum in a repeated cross-over design. The subjects were first allowed to smoke freely and then encouraged to cut down and stop their consumption. A reduction of 31 per cent was achieved on placebo gum and of 37 per cent on the nicotine gum, even before the smokers tried to

Table 2.  Effects of "Pre-load" with Nicotine Gum or Cigarette
Smoking on Smoking Behavior*†

| | | Mode of Administration | | | |
| | | Inhalation | | Chewing Gum | |
| Variable | Dose Level: | Low | High | Low | High |
|---|---|---|---|---|---|
| Latency (min) | | 4.7 | 14.8 | 4.9 | 8.0 |
| Total puff time (sec) | | 22.0 | 15.0 | 28.0 | 14.0 |

*Abstracted from Kozlowski et al. (1975).
† N.B. Other controls were included.

curtail their smoking (Table 3). Further substantial reductions ensued when the smokers actively tried to give up. There was no difference between placebo and nicotine gums in this respect. COHb levels showed similar drops, but there the differences between placebo and active gums were significant under both conditions of usual smoking (p < 0.01) and trying to abstain (p < 0.02) (Table 3). Nicotine levels were slightly lower on placebo gum than on nicotine gum, but attained similar levels after smoking. When the subjects were trying not to smoke, nicotine levels were very much lower (p < 0.001), but differences between the two gums were again not marked. It would seem that the nicotine gum does not substantially alter the number of cigarettes smoked as compared with placebo gum, but does lessen the amount of inhalation as reflected by the COHb levels. Nicotine levels differed by only about 3 ng/ml between placebo and nicotine gum conditions, probably because 2 mg per piece content is too low to produce nicotine levels comparable to smoking (4 mg is required).

## d.  Other Manipulations

A more indirect approach has comprised alteration of nicotine excretion by manipulating urinary pH. From the data of Beckett and Triggs (1966), it can be calculated that 35 percent of administered nicotine is excreted unchanged in an acidic urine, only 1 percent in an alkaline urine, and about 5 to 10 percent if the pH is uncontrolled. Based on the presumption that urinary pH manipulations would appreciably alter nicotine concentrations in the body, Schachter and his colleagues (1977) carried out the following series of experiments.

Records were kept of the amounts smoked by 7 subjects during several 2-day periods when they were taking substantial mounts of either sodium carbonate, placebo, or ascorbic acid.

The effects of these drugs on smoking are presented in Table 4. Modest increases in smoking (p < 0.08) occurred when the urine was marginally

Table 3. Mean Values of Cigarette Consumption, COHb, and Nicotine Levels in 43 Smokers Taking Nicotine and Placebo Chewing Gum*

| | Initial Levels Before Taking Gum | Smoking as Inclined | | Trying to Stop | |
| --- | --- | --- | --- | --- | --- |
| | | Placebo Gum | Nicotine Gum | Placebo Gum | Nicotine Gum |
| Daily Cigarette Consumption | 33.3 | 23.0 | 20.9 | 3.9 | 4.1 |
| COHb (%) | 8.5 | 7.2 | 6.3 | 2.9 | 2.3 |
| Nicotine (ng/ml) | 30.1 | 24.7 | 27.4 | 7.3 | 10.7 |

* Abstracted from Russell et al. (1976b).

more acid, modest decreases (p < 0.05) when alkalinization was attempted. In a replication and extension of this study, cigarette consumption increased by one-sixth when either ascorbic acid or glutamic acid was administered. This was rather surprising, as the urinary pH dropped by only about 0.2 units.

Schachter et al. (1977) extended their observations to the effect of party-going on cigarette consumption. Social events were accompanied by a lowering of urinary pH averaging 0.4 units, and cigarette consumption rose from a mean of 27.9 to 31.2. The decrease in urinary pH is presumably due to alcohol ingestion with its subsequent metabolism to acetic acid. Whether increased smoking at parties can be attributed to lowered urinary pH and more rapid excretion of nicotine is a question that awaits further study with monitoring of plasma-nicotine levels.

The basic premise of these studies have been recently examined directly (Feyerabend and Russell, 1978). Urinary excretion of nicotine was influenced markedly by pH and the rate of urine flow, both factors being important. Plasma-nicotine concentrations were about 30 percent higher under alkaline conditions than under acidic urinary conditions, although the urinary excretion rate was 30 times as slow.

A strategy stemming directly from classical pharmacology has been the use of nicotine antagonists (Stolerman et al., 1973b). The drugs administered were mecamylamine hydrochloride, a secondary compound which readily penetrates to the brain, and pentolinium tartrate, a quarternary derivative, which hardly crosses the "blood-brain-barrier." Doses were 7.5-17.5 mg and 100-150 mg, respectively. Placebo controls were incorporated, each drug being given as a single dose. A battery of tests was administered including digit symbol substitution test, hand steadiness test, assessment of subjective state, and measurements of blood pressure and pulse rate. Smoking behavior was monitored during the testing session.

Doses of mecamylamine, presumed to block the central cholinergic actions of nicotine, were associated with a significant increase in the number

Table 4.  Mean Number of Cigarettes Smoked and Urinary pH Values While Subjects Were Taking Sodium Bicarbonate, Placebo, or Ascorbic Acid*

| | Mean No. Cigarettes | | Mean Urinary pH | |
|---|---|---|---|---|
| Drug | First Drug Day | Second Drug Day | First Drug Day | Second Drug Day |
| Bicarbonate | 37.2 | 35.7 | 6.8 | 7.4 |
| Placebo | 39.4 | 34.2 | 5.7 | 5.9 |
| Ascorbic acid | 38.4 | 42.1 | 6.2 | 5.7 |

* Abstracted from Schachter et al. (1977).

of cigarettes smoked and the number of puffs on the cigarettes (Table 5). By contrast, pentolinium tended to decrease the number smoked, reaching significant levels after the higher dose. Mecamylamine but not pentolinium tended to reduce ratings of smoking satisfaction. Mecamylamine and pentolinium impaired performance on the digit symbol substitution test. Hand steadiness was improved by mecamylamine quite substantially, but pentolinium had no effect. The cardiovascular measures, introduced as a check that physiological effects were being exerted, showed the expected changes—hypotension and tachycardia—after mecamylamine administration, but pentolinium yielded no clear-cut changes. Again, although it is interesting and sure to foster further research, this study is difficult to interpret in the absence of pharmacokinetic data from monitoring of nicotine concentrations in the body. Chronic dosage would also be a useful development.

## 3. Nicotine Yield and Smoking Behavior

A commonly used approach has been to attempt to manipulate smoking by altering the amount of nicotine in the cigarette. From what has been discussed already, it will be appreciated that the nicotine yield can be a very poor indicator of the amount of nicotine extracted from the smoke and of plasma (and presumably brain) nicotine levels. Thus, number of cigarettes smoked, butt length, and nicotine content may be inaccurate estimates of nicotine delivery. Puff frequency and depth are better, but still fall short of the ideal. With these reservations in mind, some studies on manipulating nicotine yield and observing behavior are briefly reviewed.

An early study is also one of the more interesting from the point of view of nicotine delivery (Finnegan et al., 1945). Naturally low-content nicotine tobacco was treated with additional nicotine, and both low-content and

Table 5.  Mean Number of Cigarettes Smoked and Puffs on Cigarettes During 2h Test Sessions After Drug Administration*

|                |        |     | Cigarettes After | | Puffs After | |
| -------------- | ------ | --- | ----- | ------- | ----- | ------- |
| Drug Treatment | (mg)   | No. | Drug  | Placebo | Drug  | Placebo |
| Mecamylamine   | 7.5    | 8   | 4.4†  | 3.4     | 38.1  | 30.4    |
|                | 12.5   | 14  | 4.8†  | 3.2     | 36.9† | 26.1    |
|                | 17.5   | 10  | 3.8   | 3.4     | 36.6  | 32.8    |
| Pentolinium    | 100.0  | 10  | 3.6   | 3.8     | 32.9  | 35.4    |
|                | 150.0  | 10  | 3.3†  | 4.3     | 36.6  | 37.5    |

*Abstracted from Stolerman et al. (1973).
† p < 0.05.

"spiked" tobacco were made up into cigarettes yielding 0.34 and 1.96 mg nicotine per cigarette. The latter was about normal for the time of the study. Twenty-four habitual cigarette smokers smoked their usual brands for a month to establish base-line cigarette consumption. They were then switched to the added nicotine cigarettes for about 2 weeks to accustom them to the rather inferior aroma and, taste, and then for 4 weeks on the low-nicotine cigarettes, with a final 2 weeks or so on the added nicotine preparation. The degree to which nicotine was missed was assessed by questioning and ranged from none to definite and prolonged lack of satisfaction with low-nicotine cigarettes. The results are summarized in Table 6. Although the smokers who increased their consumption when switched to low-nicotine cigarettes apparently avoided dissatisfaction, it can be seen that the increase was far too small to maintain nicotine intake, unless the pattern of smoking and inhalation changed profoundly. Indeed, re-analysis of the published data shows that even the modest increase recorded was not really significant. The authors emphasize the protean nature of the smoking habit: in some smokers, nicotine becomes a major factor; in others it seems irrelevant.

A similar conclusion can be drawn from the work of Cherry and Forbes (1972). On the basis of the butt analysis of nicotine, they reported that most smokers took in less nicotine when smoking a low-nicotine brand (yield 0.77 mg) rather than a higher-nicotine brand (1.35 mg). However, a "minority" of smokers took in equal amounts of nicotine on both brands.

The smoking behavior of 36 volunteer subjects with two types of cigarettes was noted (Ashton and Watson, 1970). The low-nicotine cigarette had a filter-tip so that only 1.0 mg of nicotine was emitted in the smoke. The high-nicotine cigarette yielded 2.1 mg. The subjects undertook two driving stimulator tasks, easy and difficult, and smoked $2\frac{1}{2}$ cigarettes during the task and during a rest period afterwards. The puff frequency was noted, and the cigarette stubs were analyzed for nicotine content, allowing an estimate of the nicotine presented to the individual. During both tasks and the rest period, the puffs per minute and the time taken to smoke one cigarette were significantly different for the subjects on the two types of cigarette. The nicotine delivered to the subject, however, was a little higher on the high-nicotine cigarette, but only reached significance during the difficult task (Table 7). These data seem to strongly support the hypothesis that smokers adjust their smoking rate and pattern to maintain constant nicotine intake, but it should be pointed out that the subjects were instructed to smoke at set times.

Similar conclusions can be drawn from Frith's (1971) experiment. Nine subjects smoked three types of cigarettes delivering 1.0, 1.4, and 2.1 mg of nicotine, respectively. The rate of puffing and volume per puff were registered on a special puffing machine over an 8-hour period. The number of cigarettes smoked decreased with increase in nicotine content, and the

Table 6. Effect of Nicotine Yield on Cigarette Consumption and Smoking Satisfaction*

| Degree to Which Nicotine was Missed | Yield(Mg): | Average Daily Consumption | | | |
|---|---|---|---|---|---|
| | | Standard Brand 2.00 | Nicotine Added (First Period) 1.96 | Low Nicotine (Second Period) 0.34 | Nicotine Added 1.96 |
| Nil | N=6 | 26.90 | 26.60 | 30.90 | 26.80 |
| Mild Dissatisfaction | N=6 | 22.40 | 22.00 | 26.50 | 23.90 |
| Definite Temporary | N=3 | 23.60 | 28.30 | 28.60 | 27.60 |
| Definite Prolonged | N=9 | 25.00 | 24.70 | 24.60 | 24.90 |

* Abstracted from Finnegan et al. (1945).

## Table 7. Effect of Nicotine Content of Cigarettes on Some Smoking Variables During Two Tasks and a Rest Period*

| Type of Cigarette | Puffs per Minute | | | Time per Cigarette(min) | | Nicotine Delivery (mg) | | |
|---|---|---|---|---|---|---|---|---|
| | Easy | Difficult | Rest | Easy | Difficult | Easy | Difficult | Rest |
| Low Nicotine N=17 | 1.74 | 1.87 | 2.44 | 7.58 | 7.58 | 173 | 179 | 214 |
| | § | † | § | † | † | N.S. | † | N.S. |
| High Nicotine N=19 | 0.98 | 1.02 | 1.94 | 9.11 | 8.89 | 179 | 184 | 222 |

* Abstracted from Ashton and Watson (1970).

† p < 0.05
‡ p < 0.01
§ p < 0.001

time per cigarette increased. The subjects reported the high-nicotine cigarette to be stronger than the other two, but were unable to distinguish between the latter.

The complexities of analyzing smoking behavior are well exemplified by the study of Turner et al. (1974). Ten volunteers smoked medium-nicotine (1.4 mg) cigarettes for a week and then switched to low nicotine (0.8 mg) for the following week; the third week, they smoked very low-nicotine (0.3 mg) cigarettes. Cigarette consumption, COHb percentage, butt lengths, and nicotine contents were measured. The number of cigarettes smoked daily rose with the switch to low-nicotine cigarettes, but rose no further when very low-nicotine cigarettes were substituted (Table 8). COHb levels did not alter from medium- to low-nicotine cigarette periods, but dropped significantly when on the very low-nicotine cigarettes. The measured/expected filter nicotine ratio rose as the nicotine content dropped, indicating greater extraction of nicotine from the cigarette, and butt lengths were shorter. Six subjects found the medium brand too strong; eight initially rated the low-nicotine brand too mild; but by the end of the week, all found them acceptable. All subjects rated the very low-nicotine cigarettes weak and unsatisfying. From the calculated nicotine presentation per cigarette, it can be estimated that in order to maintain constant nicotine intake, an increase in daily consumption to 38 and 135 cigarettes, respectively, would have been required. Instead, the daily nicotine intake dropped a little on the low-nicotine cigarette and substantially on the very low one.

Jarvik's group has carried out several studies in which cigarette lengths have been altered. In one study (Goldfarb and Jarvik, 1972), 18 subjects

Table 8.   Effect of Nicotine Content of Cigarettes on Some
Smoking Variables During Ad Libitum Smoking*

| Variables | Medium | Low | Very Low |
|---|---|---|---|
| Machine-smoked yield (mg) | 1.40 | 0.80 | 0.30 |
| Daily cigarette consumption | 25.70 | 30.90 | 29.20 |
| COHb percentage | 6.34 | 6.25 | 3.80 |
| Ratio of measured nicotine butt content in study to that after machine smoking | 0.62 | 0.77 | 1.23 |
| Butt length (mm) | 8.84 | 7.20 | 4.54 |
| Calculated nicotine presentation per cigarette (mg) | 0.89 | 0.60 | 0.17 |
| Calculated nicotine presentation per day (mg) | 22.90 | 19.20 | 5.00 |
| Number of cigarettes required to maintain daily presentation | – | 38.00 | 135.00 |

*Abstracted from Turner et al. (1974).

smoked cigarettes cut to half the original length for a week, and for a second week smoked the distal half of regular length cigarettes down to a mark. The average number of the half-cigarettes smoked by the group as a whole did not differ from the number of whole cigarettes smoked in control weeks. However, 12 of the subjects did increase the number of half-cigarettes by an average of 7 per day and of the marked cigarettes by 5 per day, suggesting some attempt at compensation. The support for the titration of nicotine hypothesis is, however, very weak.

In a further study (Jarvik et al., 1978), 28 subjects were given full- half-, quarter-, and eighth-length cigarettes in random order to smoke through a puffing device for 2-hour sessions. As Table 9 shows, the number of cigarettes rises, the number of puffs decreases, and satisfaction ratings drop as the cigarette length is decreased. The peculiar distribution of the number of puffs is unexplained and the problems of estimating nicotine presentation make this study difficult to interpret. Although some partial compensation for nicotine content decrease has occurred, it is much less than the proportional decrease in cigarette length.

In the second part of this study, cigarette length and nicotine content were manipulated independently. Two strengths of cigarette, 2.0 and 0.2 mg, were smoked either full-length or quarter-length. Subjects smoked and puffed significantly more on the low-nicotine than on the high-nicotine cigarettes (Table 10). Subjects smoked significantly more quarter-length than full-length cigarettes, but did not puff more. The number of puffs per cigarette was unaffected by nicotine content. Satisfaction ratings were surprisingly unaffected. Thus, again although there was some attempt to regulate nicotine intake, it fell far short of complete compensation, the number of cigarettes smoked with the low-nicotine content increasing by only 20 percent instead of by 10 times.

As nicotine and tar contents of cigarettes are closely related, tar could

**Table 9.   Effect of Cigarette Size and Nicotine Content on Some Smoking Variables During a 2h Session\***

| Variable | Cigarette Length: | High (2mg) | | Low (0.2mg) | |
|---|---|---|---|---|---|
| | | 1 | ¼ | 1 | ¼ |
| Number of cigarettes | | 5.7 | 11.7 | 7.0 | 14.0 |
| Number of puffs | | 50.7 | 40.3 | 58.8 | 49.9 |
| Puffs/cigarette | | 8.9 | 3.4 | 8.4 | 3.6 |
| Satisfaction rating | | 3.6 | 4.0 | 3.7 | 3.9 |

\*Abstracted from Jarvik et al. (1978).

Table 10.   Effect of Cigarette Size on Some Smoking
Variables During a 2h Session*

| Variable | Cigarette Length:   1 | $^1/_2$ | $^1/_4$ | $^1/_8$ |
|---|---|---|---|---|
| Number of cigarettes | 5.4 | 8.2 | 10.3 | 15.2 |
| Number of puffs | 54.0 | 53.7 | 43.8 | 43.7 |
| Puffs/cigarette | 9.7 | 6.5 | 4.2 | 2.9 |
| Satisfaction rating | 5.2 | 4.9 | 3.6 | 2.7 |

*Abstracted from Jarvik et al. (1978).

conceivably be the important factor in regulating smoking behavior, the apparent effect of nicotine being artefactual. However, in one experiment, tar and nicotine contents were to some extent manipulated independently (Goldfarb et al., 1976). The number of cigarettes smoked per day was unaffected by tar content, whereas it decreased with increase in nicotine level; as with so many of these studies, this increase was insufficient to maintain constant nicotine intake. The smokers detected differences in the "strength" of the cigarettes, depending on nicotine and not tar content, but no systematic changes in "satisfaction" ratings were apparent.

## 4.   Nicotine and Arousal

Nicotine has a wide range of physiological actions, including a decrease in skeletal muscle tone, delay in gastric emptying, stimulation of salivary secretion, and catecholamine release with ensuing secondary effects. Plasma cortisol and growth-hormone concentrations are increased. Noradrenaline is released from peripheral noradrenergic endings. There is no evidence either supporting or refuting the hypothesis that one or more of such effects underlie the maintenance of smoking behavior.

At a psychophysiological level, several attempts have been made to interpret the maintenance of smoking behavior (see Warburton and Wesnes, 1978). In an attempt to relate patterns of smoking with personality types, Eysenck (1963) takes the view, for example, that individuals with extra-verted personalities smoke in order to increase their level of arousal. These speculations are, however, based upon the assumption that extraversion and cortical arousal bear a recognizable relationship to each other. The concept of arousal can only be applied within narrow limits when physiological measures are involved. Furthermore, nicotine and smoking effects may involve the very physiological measures used as indicators of arousal.

Of several studies in this area, the most sophisticated, and the one that brings us full circle to the opening section on why people smoke, is that of Myrsten and co-workers (1975). A questionnaire was constructed which enables smokers to be divided into those who smoke primarily in high-arousal situations—the presumption being that smoking is relaxing—and those who smoke mainly in low-arousal situations—to combat boredom or to maintain alertness. Sixteen subjects, 8 high- and 8 low-arousal smokers, were selected from the 90 male light smokers screened. Two test conditions were used: a vigilance task, which would induce low arousal; and a complex sensorimotor response task, requiring high alertness. Smoking two cigarettes during the test improved performance in the low-arousal test in the low-arousal smokers, but slightly impaired it in the high-arousal smokers. In the high-arousal test, smoking had no effect in the low-arousal smokers, but improved performance in the other group. Subjective reports tended to corroborate these differential effects of smoking in different types of smokers doing different tasks. Nevertheless, such experiments are capable of very complex interpretations when the relationship between performance is entered into the equation. This relationship follows the classical inverted-U-shaped curve (Yerkes-Dodson Law). Accordingly, several arousal points must be studied, because with only two, it is impossible to say whether the performance/arousal points are on the ascending or descending limbs of the curve. Such a study would throw much light on arousal/smoking relationships, but even so, smokers may smoke for different reasons at different times.

Among similar experiments, one other may be mentioned. Fuller and Forrest (1973) reported that heavy smokers tend to puff more on their cigarettes under low-arousal than high-arousal conditions. However, nicotine extraction from the cigarettes was not altered, suggesting perhaps that the behavioral but not the pharmacological factors could be manipulated by altering arousal conditions. This accords with the nicotine substitution studies detailed earlier, which suggested that cigarette smoking was rather more than just nicotine manipulation.

In spite of the widespread prevalence of the tobacco smoking habit and its continuing medical, commercial, and political importance, research into the psychopharmacology of nicotine and other possible important constituents of tobacco has advanced relatively slowly. In this review, we have paid particular attention to the pharmacological approach and to methodological issues as they apply to nicotine in tobacco smoking. The discussion of individual (constitutional) and environmental factors, which may modify the putative reinforcing actions of nicotine in man, has been intentionally restricted as this is a full topic in its own right. In summary, very little is known about the nature of the pharmacological rewards that are sought by novice smokers or about the maintenance of the habit in established smokers. Similarly, the physiological changes that facilitate relapse in abstaining smokers also remain obscure.

# D. REFERENCES

Alderdice, M.T., and Weiss, G.B. (1975). Effects of pharmacological agents on ($^{14}$C)-nicotine distribution and movements in slices from different rat brain areas. *Neuropharmacol.* 14:811-817.

Armitage, A.K. (1978). The role of nicotine in the tobacco smoking habit, in *Smoking Behavior*. R.E. Thornton, ed. Churchill Livingstone, Edinburgh. pp. 229-243.

Armitage, A.K., and Hall, G.H. (1968). Nicotine, smoking, and cortical activation. *Nat.* 219:1179-1180.

Armitage, A.K., Hall, G.H., and Morrison, C.F. (1968). Pharmacological basis for the tobacco smoking habit. *Nat.* 217:331-334.

Armitage, A.K., Hall, G.H., and Sellers, C.M. (1969). Effects of nicotine on electrocortical activity and acetylcholine release from the cat cerebral cortex. *Brit. J. Pharmacol.* 35:152-160.

Ashton, H., and Telford, R. (1973). Smoking and carboxyhaemoglobin. *Lancet.* 2:857-858.

Ashton, H., and Watson, D.W. (1970). Puffing frequency and nicotine intake in cigarette smokers. *Brit. Med. J.* 3:679-681.

Balfour, D.J.K. (1973). Effects of nicotine on the uptake and retention of noradrenaline and 5-hydroxytryptamine by rat brain homogenates. *Eur. J. Pharmacol.* 23:19-26.

Balfour, D.J., and Morrison, C.F. (1975). A possible role for the pituitary adrenal system in the effects of nicotine on avoidance behaviour. *Pharmacol. Biochem. Behav.* 3:349-354.

Balfour, D.J., Khullar, A.K., and Longden, A. (1975). Effects of nicotine on plasma corticosterone and brain amines in stressed and unstressed rats. *Pharmacol. Biochem. Behav.* 3:179-184.

Bättig, K., Driscoll, P., Schlalter, J., and Uster, H.J. (1976). Effects of nicotine on the exploratory locomotion patterns of female Roman high- and low-avoidance rats. *Pharmacol. Biochem. Behav.* 4:435-439.

Beckett, A.H., and Triggs, E.J. (1966). Determination of nicotine and its metabolite, cotinine, in urine by gas chromatography. *Nat.* 211:1415-1417.

Beckett, A.H., and Triggs, E.J. (1967). Enzyme induction in man caused by smoking. *Nat.* 216:587.

Beckett, A.H., Garrod, J.W., and Jenner, P. (1971). The effect of smoking on nicotine metabolism *in vivo* in man. *J. Pharm. Pharmacol.* 23:62S-67S.

Bhagat, B. (1970a). Effects of chronic administration of nicotine on storage and synthesis of noradrenaline in rat brain. *Brit. J. Pharmacol.* 38:86-92.

Bhagat, B. (1970b). Influence of chronic administration of nicotine on the turnover and metabolism of noradrenaline in the rat brain. *Psychopharmacologia.* 18:325-332.

Bhagat, B., Bayer, T., and Lind, C. (1971). Effects of chronic administration of nicotine on drug-induced hypnosis in mice. *Psychopharmacologia.* 21:287-293.

Bhattacharya, I.C., and Goldstein, L. (1970). Influence of acute and chronic nicotine administration on intra- and inter-structural relationships of the electrical activity in the rabbit brain. *Neuropharmacol.* 9:109-118.

Bovet, D., Bovet-Nitti, F., and Oliverio, A. (1966). Effects of nicotine on avoidance conditioning of inbred strains of mice. *Psychopharmacologia.* 10:1-5.

Bovet, D., Bovet-Nitti, F., and Oliverio, A. (1967). Action of nicotine on spontaneous and acquired behaviour in rats and mice. *Ann. N.Y. Acad. Sci.* 142:261-267.

Bovet-Nitti, F., and Bovet, D. (1966). Different action of nicotine during the day and night in spontaneous activity (running activity) of the rat. *Comp. Rend. Acad. Sci.* 262:316—320.

Bradley, P.B., and Elkes, J. (1957). The effect of some drugs on the electrical activity of the brain. *Brain.* 80:77-117.

Brantmark, B., Ohlin, P., and Westling, H. (1973). Nicotine-containing chewing gum as an anti-smoking aid. *Psychopharmacologia.* 31:191-200.

*British Medical Journal* (Editorial) (1977). Do people smoke for nicotine. 2:1041-1042.

Brown, D.A., and Fumagalli, L. (1977). Dissociation of α-bungarotoxin binding and receptor block in the rat superior cervical ganglion. *Brain Res.* 129:165.

Castleden, C.M., and Cole, P.V. (1974). Variations in carboxyhaemoglobin levels in smokers. *Brit. Med. J.* 4:736-738.

Cherry, W.H., and Forbes, W.F. (1972). Canadian studies aimed toward a less harmful cigarette. *J. Nat. Cancer Inst.* 48:1765-1773.

Clark, M.S. (1969). Self-administered nicotine solutions preferred to placebo by the rat. *Brit. J. Pharmacol.* 35:367P.

Crow, T.J., and Deakin, J.F.W. (1978). Brain reinforcement centers and psychoactive drugs, in *Research Advances in Alcohol and Drug Problems.* Y. Israel., F.B. Glaser, H. Kalant, R.E. Popham, W. Schmidt, and R.G. Smart, eds. Plenum Press, New York. pp. 25-76.

De Belleroche, J., and Bradford, H.F. (1978). Biochemical evidence for the presence of presynaptic receptors on dopaminergic nerve terminals. *Brain Res.* 142:53-68.

Deneau, G.A., and Inoki, R. (1967). Nicotine self-administration in monkeys. *Ann. N. Y. Acad. Sci.* 142:277-279.

Domino, E.F. (1967). Electroencephalographic and behavioural arousal effects of small doses of nicotine: A neuropsychopharmacological study *Ann. N.Y. Acad. Sci.* 142:216-244.

Domino, E.F. (1973). Neuropsychopharmacology of nicotine and tobacco smoking, in *Smoking Behaviour: Motives and Incentives.* W.L. Dunn, ed. V.H. Winston, Washington D.C. pp. 5-31.

Domino, E.F., and Lutz, M.P. (1973). Tolerance to the effects of daily nicotine on rat bar pressing behaviour for water reinforcement. *Pharmacol. Biochem. Behav.* 1:445-448.

Domino, E.F., and Olds, M.E. (1972). Effects of d-amphetamine, scopolamine, chlordiazepoxide, and diphenylhydantoin on self-stimulation behaviour and brain acetylcholine. *Psychopharmacologia.* 23:1-16.

Duggan, A.W., Hall, J.G., and Lee, C.Y. (1976). Alpha-bungarotoxin, cobra neurotoxin, and excitation of Renshaw cells by acetylcholine. *Brain Res.* 107:166-170.

Eddy, N.B., et al. (1964). Evaluation of dependence-producing drugs, W.H.O. Technical Report No. 287. World Health Organization. Geneva.

Eysenck, H.J. (1963). Personality and cigarette smoking. *Life Sci.* 3:777-792.

Fernö, O., Lichtneckert, S.J.A., and Lundgren, C.E.G. (1973). A substitute for tobacco smoking. *Psychopharmacologia.* 31:201-204.

Feyerabend, C., and Russell, M.A.H. (1978). Effect of urinary pH and nicotine excretion rate on plasma nicotine during cigarette smoking and chewing nicotine gum. *Brit. J. Clin. Pharmacol.* 5:293-298.

Feyerabend, C., Levitt, T., and Russell, M.A.H. (1975). A rapid gas-liquid chromatographic estimation of nicotine in biological fluids. *J. Pharm. Pharmacol.* 27:434-436.

Finnegan, J.K., Larson, P.S., and Haag, H.B. (1945). The role of nicotine in the cigarette habit. *Sci.* 102:94-96.

Friedman, J., Horvath, T., and Meares, R. (1974). Tobacco smoking and a "stimulus barrier." *Nat.* 248:455-456.

Frith, C.D. (1971). The effect of varying the nicotine content of cigarettes on human smoking behaviour. *Psychopharmacologia.* 19:188-192.

Fuller, R.G.C., and Forrest, D.W. (1973). Behavioural aspects of cigarette smoking in relation to arousal level. *Psycholog. Rep.* 33:115-121.

Garg, M. (1969a). Variation in effects of nicotine in four strains of rats. *Psychopharmacologia.* 14:432-438.

Garg, M. (1969b). The effect of nicotine on two different types of learning. *Psychopharmacologia.* 15:408-414.

German, D.C., and Bowden, D.M. (1974). Catecholamine systems as the neural substrate for intracranial self-stimulation: A hypothesis. *Brain Res.* 73:381-419.

Giorguieff, M.F., Le Floc'h, M.L., Westfall, T.C., Glowinski, J., and Besson, M.J. (1976). Nicotinic effect of acetylcholine on the release of newly synthesised ($^3$H) dopamine in rat striatal slices and cat caudate nucleus. *Brain Res.* 106:117–131.

Glick, S.D., Jarvik, M.E., and Nakamura, R.K. (1970). Inhibition by drugs of smoking behaviour in monkeys. *Nat.* 227:969–971.

Goldfarb, T., Gritz, E.R., Jarvik, M.E., and Stolerman, I.P. (1976). Reactions to cigarettes as a function of nicotine and "tar." *Clin. Pharmacol. Therapeut.* 19:767–772.

Goldfarb, T.L., and Jarvik, M.E. (1972). Accommodation to restricted tobacco smoke intake in cigarette smokers. *Int. J. Addict.* 7:559–565.

Goodman, F.R. (1974). Effects of nicotine on distribution and release of $^{14}$C-norepinephrine and $^{14}$C-dopamine in rat brain striatum and hypothalamus slices. *Neuropharmacol.* 13:1025–1032.

Hall, G.H., and Morrison, C.F. (1973). New evidence for a relationship between smoking, nicotine dependence, and stress. *Nat.* 243:199–201.

Hall, G.H., and Turner, D.M. (1972). Effects of nicotine on the release of $^3$H-noradrenaline from the hypothalamus. *Biochem. Pharmacol.* 21:1829–1838.

Hatchell, P.C., and Collins, A.C. (1977). Influences of genotype and sex on behavioural tolerance to nicotine in mice. *Pharmacol. Biochem. Behav.* 6:25–30.

Herxheimer, A., Griffiths, R.L., Hamilton, B., and Wakefield, M. (1967). Circulatory effects of nicotine aerosol inhalations and cigarette smoking in man. *Lancet.* 2:754–755.

Hirschhorn, I.D., and Rosecrans, S.A. (1974). Studies on the time course and the effect of cholinergic and adrenergic receptor blockers on the stimulus effect of nicotine. *Psychopharmacol.* 40:109–120.

Hubbard, J.E., and Gohd, R.S. (1975). Tolerance development to the arousal effects of nicotine. *Pharmacol. Biochem. Behav.* 3:471–476.

Hunt, S.P., and Schmidt, J. (1978). The electron microscopic autoradiographic localisation of α-bungarotoxin binding sites within the central nervous system of the rat. *Brain Res.* 142:152–159.

Hutchinson, R.R., and Emley, G.S. (1973). Effects of nicotine on avoidance, conditioned suppression, and aggression response measures in animals and man, in *Smoking Behaviour: Motives and Incentives.* W.L. Dunn, ed. V.H. Winston, Washington D.C. pp. 171–196.

Ikard, F.F., Green, D.E., and Horn, D. (1969). A scale to differentiate between types of smokers as related to the management of affect. *Int. J. Addict.* 4:649–659.

Isaac, P.F., and Rand, M.J. (1972). Cigarette smoking and plasma levels of nicotine. *Nat.* 236:308–310.

Jaffe, J.H., and Jarvik, M.E. (1978). Tobacco use and tobacco use disorder, in *Psychopharmacology: A Generation of Progress.* M.A. Lipton, A. Di Mascio, and K.F. Killam, eds. Raven Press, New York. pp. 1665–1676.

Jarvik, M.E. (1967). Tobacco smoking in monkeys. *Ann. N. Y. Acad. Sci.* 142:280–294.

Jarvik, M.E., Glick, S.D., and Nakamura, R.K. (1970). Inhibition of cigarette smoking by orally administered nicotine. *Clin. Pharmacol. Therapeut.* 11:574–576.

Jarvik, M.E., Popek, P., Schneider, M.G., Bar-Weiss, V., and Gritz, E.R. (1978). Can cigarette size and nicotine content influence smoking and puffing rates? *Psychopharmacol.* 58:303.

Johnston, L.M. (1942). Tobacco smoking and nicotine. *Lancet.* 2:742.

Keenan, A., and Johnson, F.N. (1972). Development of behavioural tolerance to nicotine in the rat. *Experimentia.* 28:428–429.

Kornetsky, C., and Eliasson, M. (1969). Reticular stimulation and chlorpromazine: An animal model for schizophrenic overarousal. *Sci.* 165:1273–1274.

Kozlowski, L.T., Jarvik, M.E., and Gritz, E.R. (1975). Nicotine regulation and cigarette smoking. *Clin. Pharmacol. Therapeut.* 17:93–97.

Kumar, R., and Stolerman, I.P. (1977). Experimental and clinical aspects of drug dependence, in *Handbook of Psychopharmacology*, Vol. 7. L.L. Iversen, S.D. Iversen, and S.H. Snyder, eds. Plenum Press, New York. pp. 321-367.

Kumar, R., Cooke, E.C., Lader, M.H., and Russell, M.A.H. (1977). Is nicotine important in tobacco smoking? *Clin. Pharmacol. Therapeut.* 21:520-529.

Lader, M.H. (1978). Nicotine and smoking behaviour. *Brit. J. Clin. Pharmacol.* 5:289-292.

Lang, W.J., Latiff, A.A., McQueen, A., and Singer, G. (1977). Self-administration of nicotine with and without a food delivery schedule. *Pharmacol. Biochem. Behav.* 7:65-70.

Larson, P.S., and Silvette, H. (1961). *Tobacco: Experimental and Clinical Studies*. Williams & Wilkins, Baltimore.

Larson, P.S. and Silvette, H. (1968). *Tobacco: Experimental and Clinical Studies*. Supp. I. Williams & Wilkins, Baltimore.

Larson, P.S., and Silvette, H. (1971). *Tobacco: Experimental and Clinical Studies*. Supp. II. Williams & Wilkins, Baltimore.

Larson, P.S., and Silvette, H. (1975). *Tobacco: Experimental and Clinical Studies*, Supp. III. Williams & Wilkins, Baltimore.

Lichtensteiger, W., Felix D., Lienhart, R., and Hefti, F. (1976). A quantitative correlation between single unit activity and fluorescence intensity of dopamine neurones in zona compacta of substantia nigra, as demonstrated under the influence of nicotine and physostigmine. *Brain Res.* 117:85-103.

Lucchesi, B.R., Schuster, C.R., and Emley, G.S. (1967). The role of nicotine as a determinant of cigarette smoking frequency in man with observations of certain cardiovascular effects associated with the tobacco alkaloid. *Clin. Pharmacol. Therapeut.* 8:789-796.

Lyon, M., and Robbins, T.W. (1975). The action of central nervous system stimulant drugs: A general theory concerning amphetamine effects, in *Current Developments in Psychopharmacology*, Vol. 2. W. Essman and L. Valzelli, eds. Spectrum, New York. pp. 89-163.

Martin, B.R., Aceto, M.D., Montgomery, J.L., May, E.L., Uwaydah, I.M., and Harris, L.S. (1978). Stereospecific binding of (-) -14C nicotine to rat brain, in *Proceedings of 7th International Congress of Pharmacology*. Paris. pp. 282.

Martin, W.R., ed (1977a). *Drug Addiction I. Morphine, Sedative/Hypnotic, and Alcohol Dependence*. Springer Verlag, Berlin.

Martin, W.R., ed. (1977b). *Drug Addiction II. Amphetamine, Psychotogen, and Marihuana Dependence*. Springer Verlag, Berlin.

McKennell, A.C. (1970). Smoking motivation factors. *Brit. J. Soc. Clin. Psychol.* 9:8-22.

McNiven, N.L., Raisinghani, K.H., Patashnik, S., and Dorfman, R.I. (1965). Determination of nicotine in smokers' urine by gas chromatography. *Nat.* 208:788.

Moore, W.M., and Brady, R.N. (1977). Studies of nicotinic acetylcholine receptor protein from rat brain II partial purification. *Biochem. Biophys. Act.* 498:331-340.

Morley, B.J., Lorden, J.F., Brown, G.B., Kemp, G.E., and Bradley, R.J. (1977). Regional distribution of nicotinic acetylcholine receptors in rat brain. *Brain Res.* 134:161-166.

Morrison, C.F. (1967). Effects of nicotine on operant behaviour of rats. *Int. J. Neuropharmacol.* 6:229-240.

Morrison, C.F. (1968). The modification by physostigmine of some effects of nicotine on bar-pressing behaviour of rats. *Brit. J. Pharmacol.* 32:28-33.

Morrison, C.F., and Armitage, A.K. (1967). Effects of nicotine upon the free operant behaviour of rats and spontaneous motor activity of mice. *Ann. N. Y. Acad. Sci.* 142:268-276.

Morrison, C.F., and Lee, P.N. (1968). A comparison of the effects of nicotine and physostigmine on a measure of activity in the rat. *Psychopharmacologia*. 13:210-221.

Morrison, C.F., and Stephenson, J.A. (1969). Nicotine injections as the conditioned stimulus in discrimination learning. *Psychopharmacologia*. 15:351-360.

Morrison, C.F., and Stephenson, J.A. (1972). The occurrence of tolerance to a central depressant effect of nicotine. *Brit. J. Pharmacol.* 45:151-156.

Morrison, C.F., Goodyear, J.M., and Sellers, C.M. (1969). Antagonism by antimuscarinic and ganglion blocking drugs of some of the behavioural effects of nicotine. *Psychopharmacologia.* 15:341-350.

Münster, G. and Bättig, K. (1975). Nicotine-induced hypophagia and hypodipsia in deprived and in hypothalamically stimulated rats. *Psychopharmacologia.* 41:211-217.

Myrsten, A.-L., Andersson, K., Frankenhaeuser, M., and Elgerot, A. (1975). Immediate effects of cigarette smoking as related to different smoking habits. *Percept. Mot. Skills.* 40:515-523.

Nelsen, J.M., and Goldstein, L. (1972). Improvement of performance on an attention task with chronic nicotine treatment in rats. *Psychopharmacologia.* 26:347-360.

Nelsen, J.M., Pelley, K., and Goldstein, L. (1975). Protection by nicotine from behavioural disruption caused by reticular formation stimulation in rats. *Pharmacol. Biochem. Behav.* 3:749-754.

Newman, L.M. (1972). Effects of cholinergic agonists and antagonists on self-stimulation behaviour in the rat. *J. Comp. Physiolog. Psychol.* 79:394-413.

Olds, M.E., and Domino, E.F. (1969). Comparison of muscarinic and nicotinic cholinergic agonists on self-stimulation behaviour. *J. Pharmacol. Exper. Ther.* 166:189-204.

Pickens, R., Meisch, R.A., and Thompson, T. (1978). Drug self-administration: An analysis of the reinforcing effects of drugs, in *Handbook of Psychopharmacology, Vol. 12.* L.L. Iversen, S.D. Iversen, and S.H. Snyder, eds. Plenum Press, New York. pp. 1-37.

Pradhan, S.N., and Bowling, C. (1971). Effects of nicotine on self-stimulation in rats. *J. Pharmacol. Exper. Ther.* 176:229-243.

Pradhan, S.N., and Dutta, S.N. (1970). Comparative effects of nicotine and amphetamine on timing behaviour in rats. *Neuropharmacol.* 9:9-16.

Proc. Bayer Symposium IV. (1973). *Psychic Dependence.* L. Goldberg and H. Hoffmeister, eds. Springer Verlag, Berlin.

Proc. Symposium on Control of Drug-Taking Behaviour by Schedules of Reinforcement (1976). *Pharmacolog. Rev.* 27:291-446.

Rosecrans, J.A. (1971). Effects of nicotine on behavioural arousal and brain 5-hydroxytryptamine function in female rats selected for differences in activity. *Eqr. J. Pharmacol.* 14:29-37.

Rosecrans, J.A., and Chance, W.T. (1977). Cholinergic and non-cholinergic aspects of the discriminative stimulus properties of nicotine, in *Discriminative Stimulus Properties of Drugs.* H. Lal, ed. Plenum Press, New York. pp. 155-185.

Rosenthal, R.N., and Slotkin, T.A. (1977). Development of nicotinic responses in the rat adrenal medulla and long-term effects of neonatal nicotine administration. *Brit. J. Pharmacol.* 60:59-64.

Rottenstein, H., Pierce, G., Russ, E., Felder, D., and Montgomery, H. (1960). Influence of nicotine on the blood flow of resting skeletal muscle and of the digits in normal subjects. *Ann. N. Y. Acad. Sci.* 90:102-113.

Routtenberg, A. (1968). The two-arousal hypothesis: Reticular formation and limbic system. *Psycholog. Rev.* 75:51-80.

Russell, M.A.H. (1977). Smoking problems: An overview, in *Research on Smoking Behaviour.* M.E. Jarvik, J.W. Cullen, E.R. Gritz, T.M. Vogt, and L.J. West, eds. NIDA Research Monograph No. 17, U.S. Government Printing Office, Washington, D.C. pp. 13-34.

Russell, M.A.H., and Feyerabend, C. (1978). Cigarette smoking: A dependence on high-nicotine boli. *Drug Metab. Revs.* 8:29-57.

Russell, M.A.H., Wilson, C., Cole, P.V., Idle, M., and Feyerabend, C. (1973a). Comparison of increases in carboxyhaemoglobin after smoking "extra mild" and "non-mild" cigarettes. *Lancet.* 2:687-690.

Russell, M.A.H., Wilson, C., Patel, U.A., Cole, P.V., and Feyerabend, C. (1973b). Comparison of effect on tobacco consumption and carbon monoxide absorption of changing to high- and low-nicotine cigarettes. *Brit. Med. J.* 4:512-516.

Russell, M.A.H., Peto, J., and Patel, U.A. (1974). The classification of smoking by factorial structure of motives. *J. Roy. Stat. Soc.* 137:313-333.

Russell, M.A.H., Cole, P.V., Idle, M.S., and Adams, L. (1975a). Carbon monoxide yields of cigarettes and their relation to nicotine yield and type of filter. *Brit Med. J.* 3:71-73.

Russell, M.A.H., Wilson, C., Patel, U.A., Feyerabend, C., and Cole, P.V. (1975b). Plasma nicotine levels after smoking cigarettes with high-, medium-, and low-nicotine yields. *Brit. Med. J.* 2:414-416.

Russell, M.A.H., Feyerabend, C., and Cole, P.V. (1976a). Plasma nicotine levels after cigarette smoking and chewing nicotine gum. *Brit. Med. J.* 1:1043-1046.

Russell, M.A.H., Wilson, C., Feyerabend, C., and Cole, P.V. (1976b). Effect of nicotine chewing gum on smoking behaviour and as an aid to cigarette withdrawal. *Brit. Med. J.* 2:391-393.

Salvaterra, P.M., Mahler, H.R., and Moore, W.J. (1975). Subcellular and regional distribution of [125]I-labelled α-bungarotoxin binding in rat brain and its relationship to acetylcholines- terase and choline acetyltransferase. *J. Biolog. Chem.* 250:6469-6475.

Sanger, D.J. (1978). Nicotine and schedule-induced drinking in rats. *Pharmacol. Biochem. Behav.* 8:343-346.

Sanger, D.J., and Blackman, D.E. (1976). Rate-dependent effects of drugs: A review of the literature. *Pharmacol. Biochem. Behav.* 4:73-83.

Schachter, S., Silverstein, B., Kozlowski, L.T., Perlick, D., Herman, C.P., and Liebling, B. (1977). Studies of the interaction of psychological and pharmacological determinants of smoking. *J. Exper. Psychol.* 106:3-40.

Schechter, M.D., and Jellinek, P. (1975). Evidence for a cortical locus for the stimulus effect of nicotine. *Eur. J. Pharmacol.* 34:65-73.

Schechter, M.D., and Rosecrans, J.A. (1971). CNS effect of nicotine as the discriminative stimulus for the rat in a T-maze. *Life Sci.* 10:821-832.

Schechter, M.D., and Rosecrans, J.A. (1972). Behavioural tolerance to an effect of nicotine in the rat. *Arch. Int. Pharmacodyn.* 195:52-56.

Schechter, N., Handy, I.C., Pezzementi, L., and Schmidt, J. (1978). Distribution of α- bungarotoxin binding sites in the central nervous system and peripheral organs of the rat. *Toxicon.* 16:245-251.

Speth, R.C., Chen, F.M., Lindstrom, J.M., Kobayashi, R.M., and Yamamura, H.I. (1977). Nicotinic cholinergic receptors in rat brain identified by ([125]I) naja naja siamensis alpha- toxin binding. *Brain Res.* 131:350-355.

Stitzer, M., Morrison, J., and Domino E. (1970). Effects of nicotine on fixed-interval behaviour and their modification by cholinergic antagonists. *J. Pharmacol. Exper. Ther.* 171:166-177.

Stolerman, I.P., Bunker, P., and Jarvik, M.E. (1974). Nicotine tolerance in rats: Role of dose and dose interval. *Psychopharmacologia.* 34:317-324.

Stolerman, I.P., Fink, R., and Jarvik, M.E. (1973a). Acute and chronic tolerance to nicotine measured by activity in rats. *Psychopharmacologia.* 30:329-342.

Stolerman, I.P., Goldfarb, T., Fink, R., and Jarvik, M.E. (1973b). Influencing cigarette smoking with nicotine antagonists. *Psychopharmacologia.* 28:247-259.

Sulser, F., and Sanders-Bush, E. (1971). Effects of drugs on amines in the CNS. *Ann. Rev. Pharmacol.* 11:209-230.

Thompson, T., and Pickens, R., eds. (1971). *Stimulus Properties of Drugs.* Appleton-Century- Crofts, New York.

Thornton, R.E., ed. (1978). *Smoking Behaviour. Physiological and Psychological Influences.*

Churchill Livingstone, Edinburgh.

Tomkins, S.E. (1966). Psychological model for smoking behaviour. *Am. J. Pub. Health and Nation's Health.* 56:17–20.

Turner, J.A. McM., Sillett, R.W., and Ball, K.P. (1974). Some effects of changing to low-tar and low-nicotine cigarettes. *Lancet.* 2:737–739.

Ulett, J.A., and Itil, T.M. (1969). Quantitative electroencephalogram in smoking and smoking deprivation. *Sci.* 164:969–970.

Van Loon, G.R., Scapagnigni, V., Cohen, R., and Ganong, W.F. (1971). Effect of intraventricular administration of adrenergic drugs on the adrenal venous 17-hydroxycorticosteroid response to surgical stress in the dog. *Neuroendocrinol.* 8:257–272.

Vasquez, A.J., and Toman, J.E.P. (1967). Some interactions of nicotine with other drugs upon central nervous function. *Ann. N. Y. Acad. Sci.* 142:201–215.

Wanner, H.V., and Bättig, K. (1966). Wirkung von Nikotin und Amphetamin auf die Selbstreisung bei der Ratte. *Helvet. Physiolog. Pharmacolog. Acta.* 24:122–124.

Warburton, D.M., and Wesnes, K. (1978). Individual differences in smoking and attentional behaviour, in *Smoking Behaviour.* R.E. Thornton, ed. Churchill Livingstone, Edinburgh. pp. 19–43.

Weiss, G.B., and Alderdice, M.T. (1975). Characterisation of ($^{14}$C)-nicotine accumulation and movements in slices from different rat brain areas. *Neuropharmacol.* 14:265–273.

Westfall, T.C. (1974). Effect of nicotine and other drugs on the release of $^{3}$H-norepinephrine and $^{3}$H-dopamine from rat brain slices. *Neuropharmacol.* 13:693–700.

Westfall, T.C., Fleming, R.M., Fudger, M.F., and Clark, W.G. (1967). Effect of nicotine and related substances upon amine levels in the brain. *Ann. N. Y. Acad. Sci.* 142:83–100.

W.H.O. (1975). Smoking—its effect on health. World Health Organization Technical Report Series, No. 568.

Wise, R.A. (1978). Catecholamine theories of reward: A critical review. *Brain Res.* 152:215–247.

Yamamoto, K.I., and Domino, E.F. (1965). Nicotine-induced EEG and behavioural arousal. *Int. J. Neuropharmacol.* 4:359–373.

Yanagita, T., Ando, K., Oinuma, N., and Ishida, K. (1974). Intravenous self-administration of nicotine and an attempt to produce smoking behaviour in monkeys, in *Report of the 36th Annual Scientific Meeting, Committee on Problems of Drug Dependence.* National Academy of Sciences, Washington D.C. pp. 567–578.

Current Developments in Psychopharmacology, Volume 6
© 1981, Spectrum Publications, Inc.

CHAPTER 6

# THE ANTIDEPRESSANT EFFECT OF LITHIUM

ARIEL ARIELI
ELIE LEPKIFKER

## A. INTRODUCTION

Although there is almost general agreement that lithium carbonate has a clear therapeutic effect upon the manic phases of the manic-depressive illness and also a prophylactic effect against both manic and depressive relapses, its action on the depressive phase of the disease as well as on other forms of endogenic depression is still questioned. Clinicians are still reluctant to use lithium as an antidepressant drug.

Very few controlled studies have been conducted in order to verify the antidepressant action of lithium. Most of these used placebo as a control, and only three used another known antidepressant for comparison. We shall review these studies in this text, and especially the studies that compared lithium to another antidepressant agent. We shall also present for the first time the results of a study concluded in 1977 on the antidepressant effect of lithium carbonate in acute endogenous depression, as compared to clomipramine, which is a tricyclic antidepressant commonly used in Europe and Israel, and to placebo.

The importance of using these two controlled groups—necessary in our opinion in any psychopharmacological research comparing two antidepressant drugs—has been entirely proven in the present study. In view of the growing number of available antidepressant agents, the awareness toward possible side effects of these medications, and also the improved biochemical methods used in psychopharmacological research, there is an ever-increasing need to find the most appropriate medication for each given patient. It is no longer sufficient to establish that a new medication has an antidepressant effect. It is necessary to recognize its action upon the various target symptoms of depression. This also applies to lithium.

Up to now, the precise mechanisms of action of the various antidepressants, including lithium, have not been sufficiently elucidated, but attempts are being made to use biochemical characteristics for predicting response to antidepressant medications. These biochemical findings may lead to a better understanding of the mechanisms involved.

## B.  THE OVERALL ANTIDEPRESSANT EFFECT OF LITHIUM

The antidepressant effect of lithium was first tested by Cade (1949) on a small group of depressive patients, but he found no such effect. Since then, several clinical trials, controlled or uncontrolled, have been reported.

### 1.  Open Trials

Mendels (1975, 1976) reviewed nine uncontrolled studies between 1949 and 1975. Those were the studies of Cade (1949), Noack and Trautner (1951), Vojtechovsky (1957) (cited by Schou in 1968), Andreani et al. (1958), Dyson and Mendels (1968), Van der Velde (1970), Nahunek et al. (1970), Noyes et al. (1971), and Bennie (1975). The recent study of Neubauer and Bermingham (1976) should be added.

No definite conclusions should be drawn from these uncontrolled studies, especially since they cover a heterogenous population of patients including even neurotic depressive subjects. Nevertheless, in 7 of these 10 trials, lithium appeared to have a clear antidepressant effect.

### 2.  Controlled Studies

Mendels (1976) also reviewed 10 controlled studies in which a lithium-treated group was compared to a placebo group, or to a group receiving a known tricyclic antidepressant. To this review we shall add the research published by Watanabe et al. (1975), using imipramine as a control. In these 11 controlled trials, 162 hospitalized patients were studied.

#### a.  Controlled Studies with Placebo

Eight controlled studies used placebo: Hansen et al. (1968), Goodwin et al. (1969), Stokes et al. (1971), an additional publication by Goodwin et al. (1972), Noyes et al. (1974), Johnson (1974), Baron et al. (1975), and a recent report by Mendels cited in this author's review (1976) already quoted.

In two of these controlled studies with placebo, no antidepressant effect for lithium was shown. Hansen et al. (1968) used a crossover design, in which lithium was given for 2 weeks to 12 severely depressed endogenous patients and was then replaced by placebo. Only one patient suffered a relapse with placebo substitution after having improved on lithium. Some of the other patients (the exact number is not quoted) improved with lithium treatment, but suffered no relapse with placebo. Therefore, the author concluded that the effect of lithium was not specific.

Stokes et al. (1971) treated their patients with an adequate dosage of lithium during a period of 10 days. They found no significant difference between patients treated with lithium and patients given placebo.

In the 6 other studies using placebo substitution, lithium proved to be an effective antidepressant, as a significant number of patients in each of these studies responded to lithium treatment and subsequently relapsed when the drug was substituted by placebo. This effect was more obvious in bipolar depressive patients than in unipolar depressive patients.

**b. Controlled Studies with a Known Antidepressant Medication**

Fieve et al. (1968) compared 17 depressed patients who received lithium to 12 patients treated with imipramine. They evaluated their patients with the Zuckerman Multiple Affect Adjective Checklist (Zuckerman, 1960), and with the Psychiatric Evaluation Form, Depressive Scale (Spitzer et al. 1967). They found that after 2 to 3 weeks of treatment, imipramine appeared to be a moderate to strong antidepressant agent, whereas lithium showed only the mildest antidepressant effect. Unfortunately, we have no information concerning the dosage of lithium or imipramine used. We cannot therefore ascertain that effective dosages were reached.

Fieve's conclusion and their own personal impression brought Watanabe et al. (1975) to test lithium as an antidepressant only on moderately depressed patients, whereas severely depressed and especially suicidal patients were excluded. They compared 26 depressed patients receiving lithium (10 inpatients and 16 outpatients) to 19 patients treated with imipramine (5 inpatients and 14 outpatients). The patients received lithium in doses up to 900 mg per day versus a maximal dose of 150 mg of imipramine. Patients were evaluated with the Hamilton Depression Scale (Hamilton, 1960) and the Beck Self-Inventory Scale (Beck et al., 1961). The authors concluded that lithium had an antidepressant effect on moderately depressed patients, since there was no significant difference in the good overall therapeutic response to the two drugs.

Mendels et al. (1972) compared 12 patients treated with lithium to 12 patients receiving desimipramine. The maximal doses used were 1,000 to 2,000 mg of lithium per day, or 100 to 200 mg of desimipramine per day. The patients were severely endogenous-depressed patients (with an initial total Hamilton score of at least 15). The clinical evaluation was done with the Hamilton Depressive Scale (Hamilton, 1960) and with a personal inventory listing 10 cardinal symptoms. Their results showed that 9 of the 12 patients treated with lithium improved by 50 percent of the total Hamilton score, while 6 of the 12 patients receiving desimipramine showed a similar improvement. Here again, lithium proved to be an effective antidepressant. There was no significant difference between the two drugs.

## C. METHODS

### 1. Selection of Patients

The subjects of this trial were selected from patients routinely referred for hospitalization in the psychiatric open ward of the Chaim Sheba Medical Center, Tell Hashomer, Israel, by doctors in charge of the department or by other psychiatrists. Admission was restricted to endogenous-depressive patients responding to the following criteria:

1. One of the following three diagnostic categories, in accordance with the Diagnosis and Statistical Manual of Mental Disorders (American Psychiatric Association, Washington, D.C., 1968): manic depressive illness (unipolar endogenic depression), involutional depression (unipolar endogenic depression), or manic depressive illness—circular depressed (bipolar endogenic depression). Schizophrenic or neurotic depressed patients were not included.
2. At least one previous episode of depression or mania.
3. The present episode started at least 1 month prior to hospitalization.
4. No history and no signs of neurological, renal, hepatic, cardiovascular, or arteriosclerotic disorders.

The selection was made by the two researchers in agreement with at least one senior psychiatrist of the department.

### 2. Drug Administration

All patients were initially given placebo for a 1-week washing-out period. They were then assigned either lithium, clomipramine, or placebo in identical capsules for the double-blind trial. The patients were informed that they were participating in a clinical study aimed at determining the influence of lithium therapy in depression. Neither of the two psychiatrists participating in the study knew which medication was given to which patient. The

---

Worrall et al. (1979) recently published 2 randomized double-blind controlled studies. In the first, they compared the effects of lithium against imipramine in 29 female in-patients with bipolar or unipolar recurrent affective disorder. In the second, they compared a combination of lithium and tryptophan against tryptophan alone in 29 acutely depressed female in-patients. In both, lithium showed major acute antidepressant effects.

physician responsible for the trial was informed of the medication given only when severe toxic effects appeared or when the serum lithium level was higher than 1.6 mEq/liter. The method of administration of the active medication, which was maintained for 3 weeks, was as follows:

During the first week, the maximum number of capsules per day was 6, this dosage being reached progressively, generally on the fourth day. If the clinical response was not satisfactory, the dosage was increased to 8 capsules per day during the second week, and similarly to 10 per day during the third week. During the second part of the trial however, because of numerous toxic reactions, the maximum dosage remained at 6 during the second week and was increased to 8 during the third week. In case severe neurotoxicity or other toxic side effects appeared, the dosage was reduced and/or an antidote, such as an anti-Parkinsonian medication was added. The only additional medication permitted during the washing-out period as well as during the active treatment were hypnotics, either chloralhydrate (1 g), or sodium amytal (0.2 g).

### 3. Laboratory Examinations

Each patient underwent the following examinations at the end of the washing-out period, before active treatment: routine hemotological tests, liver function tests, blood glucose and urea, creatinine clearance, and also electrocardiogram (ECG) and electroencephalogram (EEG). At the end of each week of treatment, serum lithium level, urea, and creatinine clearance were measured. Whenever signs of neurotoxicity appeared, the serum lithium level was redetermined immediately.

### 4. Clinical Evaluation

At the end of the washing-out period—week 00—an additional clinical evaluation was done with the Hamilton Depressive Scale and the Clinical Global Impression. This evaluation was done separately by the two investigators, after which the scores were compared and the final score was given by consensus of the two. Only patients with a total Hamilton score of at least 14 were admitted for research.*

---

*We used the original Hamilton form, listing 21 symptoms for this evaluation. However, only 17 items were considered for statistical analysis by the Biometric Laboratory Information Processing System of the National Institute of Mental Health, since the others are not significant for factor analysis (see Hamilton, 1967). Furthermore, it appeared that item number 14 (genital symptoms) was irrelevant for our patients during their hospitalization, so that finally the total Hamilton score was based on 16 items, and the minimum score for admittance was reduced to 12. Two patients received the minimal score of 12.

## D. RESULTS

### 1. Dropouts

Of the 41 patients originally admitted to the research program, only 33 completed the trial. Of the eight patients who dropped out, seven did so during the washing-out period. In one case, the diagnosis proved to be a schizo-affective depressed state; in another, a brain tumor; the other five improved during the washing-out period to such a point that they did not meet the requirements for the study anymore. The eighth patient left during the active treatment due to lack of cooperation. One female patient (number 511) dropped out 2 days before completing the program, because of severe lithium intoxication. To avoid bias towards the lithium group, this patient was nevertheless included in that group.

### 2. Patient Characteristics

The 33 remaining patients were divided at random into 3 subgroups by the biostatistic unit of the Chaim Sheba Hospital. Group A, consisting of 12 patients, was assigned lithium; group B, consisting of 10 patients, was assigned clomipramine; group C, with 11 patients, was assigned placebo. In the entire group, there were 12 male and 21 female patients. The ages ranged from 29 to 72 years, with a mean of 50.7. Twelve patients were diagnosed recurrent unipolar endogenic depression (manic-depressive illness, depressed and involutional depression), and 11 received the diagnosis of bipolar endogenic depression (manic-depressive illness, circular depressed). The initial Hamilton score for the whole group was 21.86, ranging from 12 to 30.

Table 1 shows the distribution of patients' characteristics in the three groups. There was no significant difference between the three groups for patient characteristics, aside from the fact that in the clomipramine group, 5 of the 10 patients selected at random happened to be bipolar.

### 3. Overall Therapeutic Results and Time Lapse

#### a. Total Hamilton Score

Figure 1 illustrates the changes in total Hamilton scores, presented as the ratio sum of scores/average, calculated weekly for each of the three groups. For each group, a progressive improvement was noted from week to week, and a significant improvement ($p < 0.05$ by t-test) was obtained between the beginning and the end of the trial. However, there were differences in the significant improvements obtained with each of the three drugs in relation to the periods: In the placebo group, a significant improvement appeared only between week 00 and week 03; in the clomipra-

Table 1. Patients Characteristics

| Group | No. | Sex (M) | Sex (F) | Mean Age (Yrs) | Diagnosis Unipolar Depression — Unipolar | Diagnosis Unipolar Depression — Involutional | Bipolar Depression | Mean Initial Hamilton Score |
|---|---|---|---|---|---|---|---|---|
| A = Lithium | 12 | 4 | 8 | 52 (32–68) | 6 | 3 | 3 | 22.3 (12–29) |
| B = Clomipramine | 10 | 5 | 5 | 45.8 (29–62) | 3 | 2 | 5 | 21.3 (14–30) |
| C = Placebo | 11 | 3 | 8 | 53.5 (38–72) | 6 | 2 | 3 | 23 (12–30) |

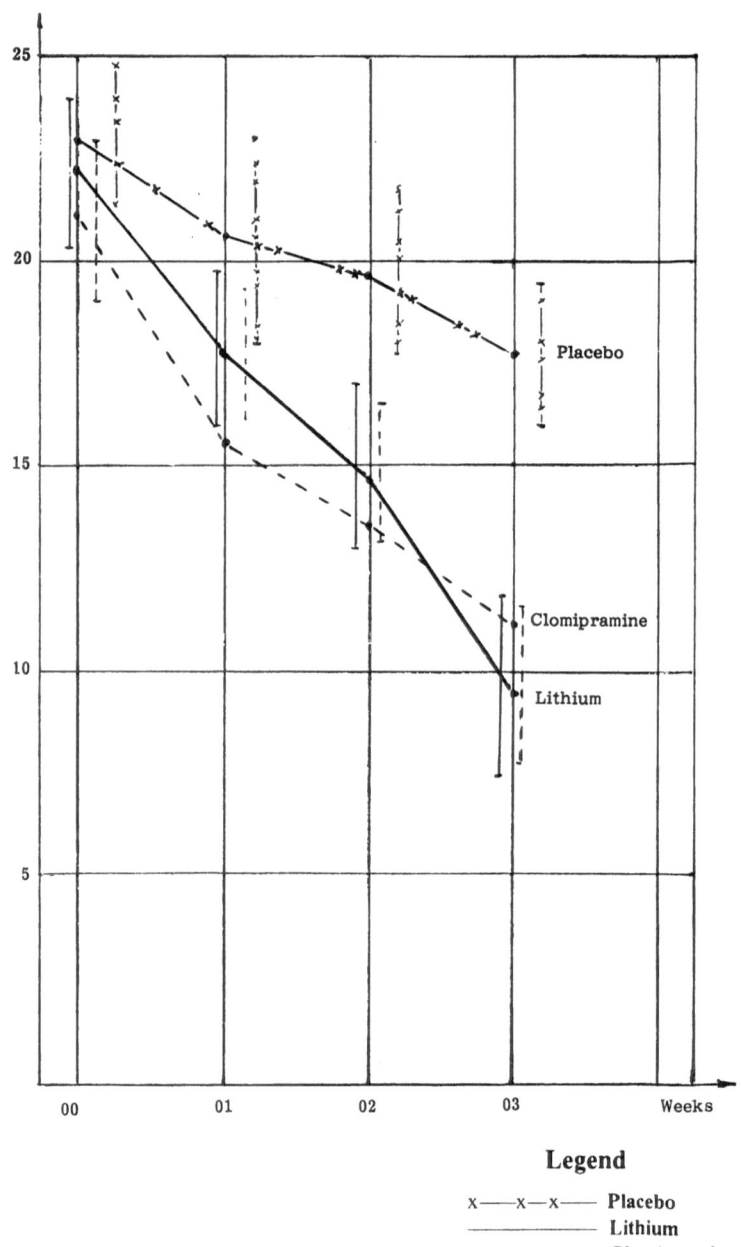

**Figure 1.** Total Hamilton Score (mean ± SE)

mine group, a significant improvement was shown between weeks 00 and 03 with some improvement between weeks 00 and 02; in the lithium group, the improvement was significant between initial and final weeks, between weeks 00 and 02, and also between weeks 02 and 03.

By comparing the three groups, we noted that the initial value for each was not statistically different. At week 02, there was a significant difference between clomipramine and placebo, also between lithium and placebo (although smaller than the difference between clomipramine and placebo), but the difference between clomipramine and lithium was not significant. At week 03, we found a significant difference between lithium and placebo, a smaller but still significant difference between clomipramine and placebo, but no significant difference between clomipramine and lithium.

The mean improvement for each group, in percentage of total Hamilton score, was as follows: lithium—56.05 percent, clomipramine—46.9 percent, placebo—23 percent.

### b. Clinical Global Impression

A significant difference in global improvement ($p < 0.05$) was found only between the lithium and placebo groups for the period from the beginning to the end of the trial. The clomipramine group showed a greater improvement than the placebo group, but the difference was not significant. There was no significant difference between clomipramine and lithium.

### 4. Factor Analysis of Hamilton Depression Scale and Time Lapse

### c. Factor I: Sleep Disturbances (Items 4,5,6)

In all 3 trial groups, including the placebo group, a significant difference was obtained between week 00 and the final week and also between week 02 and week 03 (see Figure 2A).

When comparing the 3 groups, we found no difference in the degrees of improvement at weeks 02 and 03. We noticed that for some unexplained reason, all patients of the lithium clomipramine groups showed initial values significantly lower than the placebo group.

### d. Factor II: Somatization (Items 11,12,13,15)

A significant improvement between the initial week and the final week appeared only in the lithium and clomipramine groups. In the lithium group, the improvement was also significant between weeks 02 and 03 (see Figure 2B).

When comparing the 3 groups, we noticed that during period 03, the value obtained for the placebo group did not improve and was significantly higher than for both the lithium and clomipramine groups.

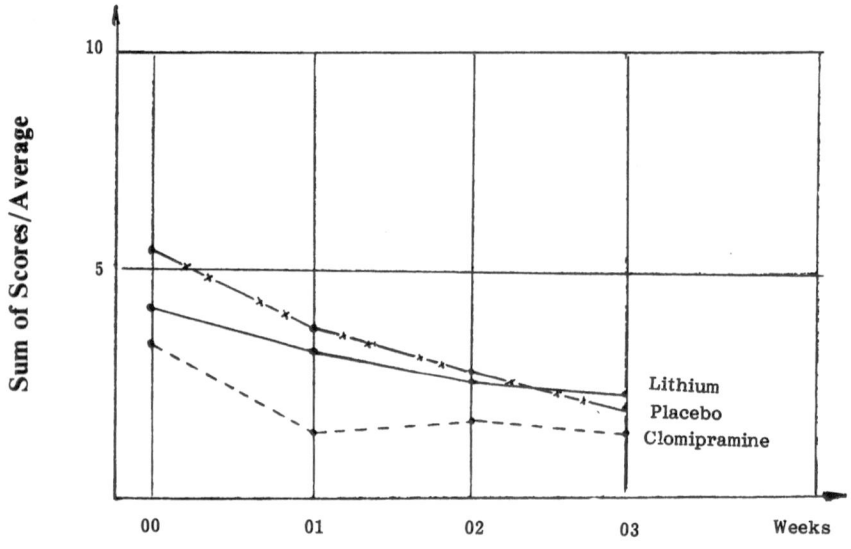

**Figure 2A.**   Sleep Disturbances.

### e. Factor III: Depression (Items 1,2,3)

A significant improvement between the initial and final weeks appeared only in the lithium and clomipramine groups. In the lithium group, the improvement was also significant between weeks 00 and 02, as well as between weeks 02 and 03. In the clomipramine group, the improvement was significant between weeks 00 and 02, but not between weeks 02 and 03 (see Figure 2C).

The comparison between the groups at week 02 showed a significant difference in the degree of improvement between lithium and placebo, and between lithium and clomipramine. The difference was not significant between clomipramine and placebo. At week 03, the difference was again significant between lithium and placebo and between lithium and clomipramine. The difference between clomipramine and placebo was also significant.

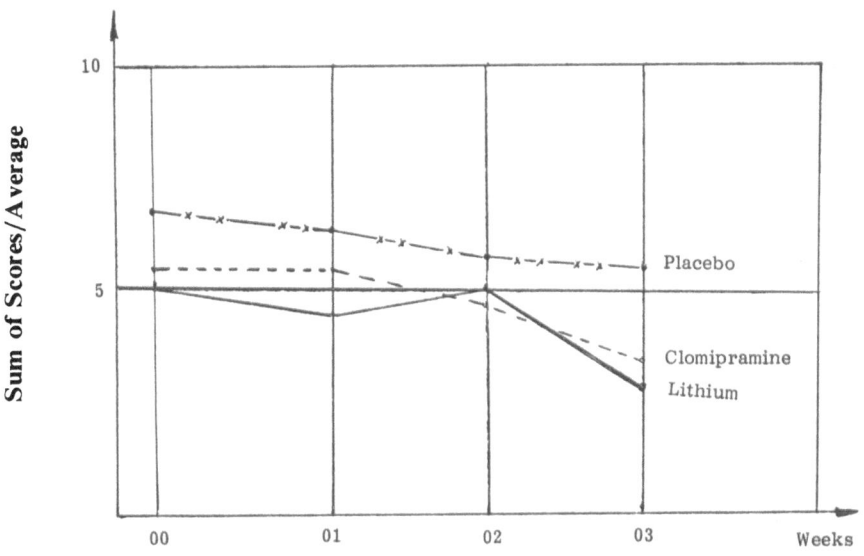

**Figure 2B.**  Somatization.

**Legend**
x——x—x——x Placebo
————————— Lithium
------------ Clomipramine

#### f. Factor IV: Apathy (Items 7,8,17)

A significant difference between the initial and final weeks appeared only in the lithium and clomipramine groups. In the clomipramine group, the improvement was already significant between weeks 00 and 02, while not yet for the lithium group (see Figure 2D).

The comparison between the groups at week 02 showed a significant difference in improvement between the clomipramine and placebo groups. At week 03, the difference became significant for both clomipramine and lithium versus placebo, but was greater with clomipramine.

#### g. Factor V: Anxiety/Agitation (Items 9,10,11)

A significant improvement between the initial and final weeks was obtained with lithium only. Between weeks 00 and 02, there was a significant improvement both in the lithium and clomipramine groups. When compar-

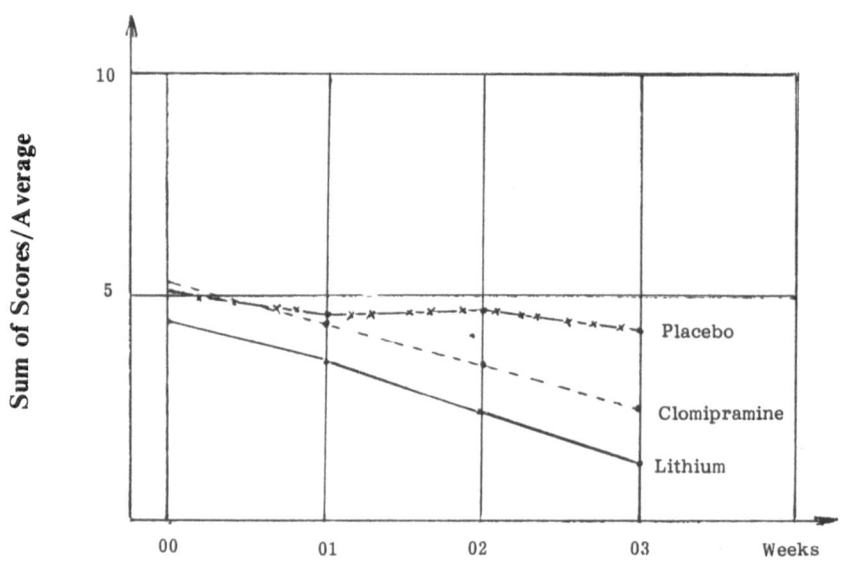

**Legend**

x——x—x——x **Placebo**

. —————— **Lithium**

**Figure 2C.**   Depression.       ------------ **Clomipramine**

ing the groups, we found a significant difference between lithium and placebo at weeks 02 and 03, while no such difference appeared between clomipramine and placebo. The difference was not significant between clomipramine and lithium, but the lithium group showed a greater improvement (see Figure 2E).

## 5.  Dosage

The total Hamilton scores revealed a greater improvement with the revised dosage than with the original one, but the difference between the two was not significant. We should stress the fact that the statistical evaluation was made difficult by the further subdivision because of the small number of patients in each group (7 versus 5).

## 6.  Unipolar Versus Bipolar Depression

Eleven of the depressed patients studied were bipolar. This was a small

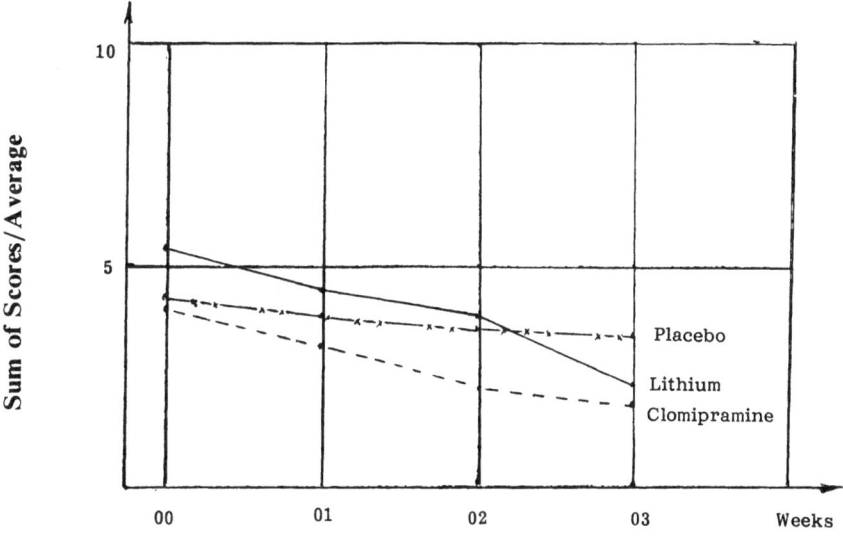

**Legend**

x——x—x——x **Placebo**
——————— **Lithium**
------------ **Clomipramine**

**Figure 2D.**  Apathy.

number for statistical assessment, especially when divided into three groups. Nevertheless, an interesting fact was noted: In the lithium as well as in the clomipramine groups, the improvement in total Hamilton score was by far superior for bipolar depressive patients than for all the patients involved in the study. While the whole group of 12 patients treated with lithium showed a mean improvement of 56.05 percent, 2 of the 3 bipolar patients improved by 86.9 and 70.8 percent, respectively. Although the mean improvement for the 10 patients concerned in the clomipramine group was 46.9 percent, 4 of the 5 bipolar patients showed an improvement of 71.4, 70.8, 73.3, and 84.0 percent, respectively (Table 2).

## 7.  Side Effects

The side effects and toxic symptoms observed in the lithium group are listed in Table 3. Seven patients received the original dosage, while five others received a revised dosage. The following statistics were also indicated for each patient: age, creatinine clearance, maximal daily dosage (mg), and

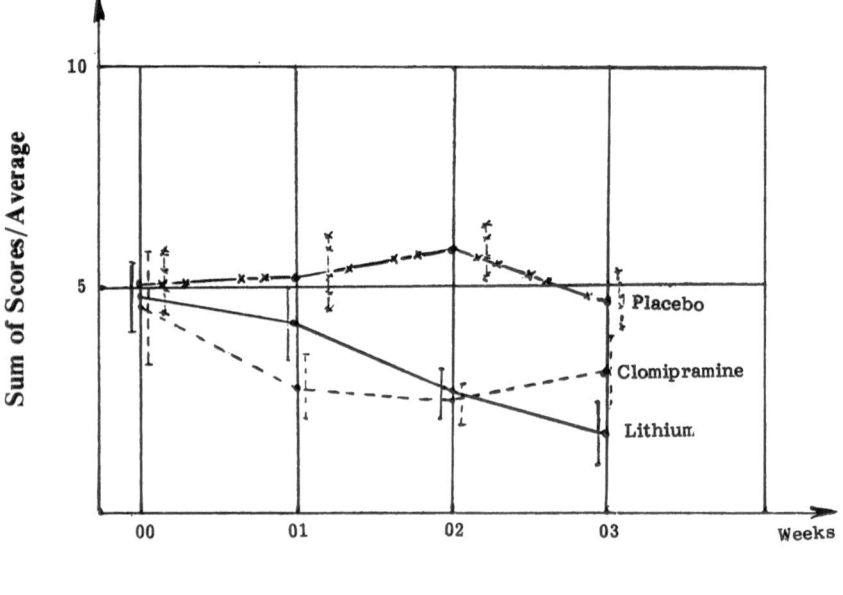

**Figure 2E.**   Anxiety/Agitation.

**Legend**

x——x—x——x **Placebo**
————————— **Lithium**
------------ **Clomipramine**

serum lithium concentration (in mEq/liter). Of the seven patients who were given the original dosage, six suffered from tremor, three from severe dizziness, two from nausea, and one from severe diarrhea. One female patient (number 511) developed a toxic confusional state and the treatment was discontinued 2 days before concluding the trial. In 2 patients, the creatinine clearance was below 70 ml/min. In all 7 patients, serum lithium levels rose above 1.0 mEq/liter, and in 3 of them, above 2.0 mEq/liter.

In the revised dosage program, only one patient out of five suffered from a severe tremor, two from dizziness (the two oldest patients of this group), and one patient complained of severe nausea; two developed no concomitant symptoms. The values of creatinine clearance remained within normal range in all cases. In 4 of these 5 patients, the serum lithium concentration did not pass 1.0 mEq/liter.

The improvement resulting from the change in the dosage program was

Table 2. Improvement in Total Hamilton Score in the 11 Bipolar Patients

| Lithium Mean for the Whole Group 56.05% | | Clomipramine Mean for the Whole Group 46.9% | | Placebo Mean for the Whole Group 23% | |
|---|---|---|---|---|---|
| Patient No. | Percent Improvement | Patient No. | Percent Improvement | Patient No. | Percent Improvement |
| 002 | 21.4 | 001 | 0.0 | 507 | 76.0 |
| 508 | 86.9 | 006 | 71.4 | 513 | -11.1 |
| 011 | 70.8 | 501 | 70.8 | 518 | 22.2 |
| | | 010 | 73.3 | | |
| | | 514 | 84.0 | | |

# Table 3. Side Effects in the Lithium Group

| A. Original Dosage N = 7 | | | | | | B. Revised Dosage N = 5 | | | | | |
| --- | --- | --- | --- | --- | --- | --- | --- | --- | --- | --- | --- |
| Patient No. | Age | Creatinine Clearance | Max. Daily Dosage (mg) | Lithium Level (mEq/liter) | Side Effects | Patient No. | Age | Creatinine Clearance | Side Effects | Max. Daily Dosage (mg) | Lithium Level (mEq/liter) |
| 002 | 53 | 108 | 2500 | 1.1 | Tremor + | 011 | 55 | 136 | Asymptomatic | 2000 | 1.0 |
| 007 | 50 | 80 | 2000 | 1.2 | Tremor ++ Dizziness ++ Vomiting + | 012 | 68 | 130 | Tremor ++ Dizziness ++ | 1500 | 1.0 |
| 502 | 64 | 104 | 1500 | 1.8 | Tremor ++ Dizziness ++ Diarrhea ++ | 519 | 35 | 109 | Nausea ++ | 1500 | 0.8 |
| 503 | 32 | 170 | 2000 | 2.95 | Tremor + Dizziness +++ Vomiting + | 520 | 45 | 130 | Asymptomatic | 2000 | 0.8 |
| 505 | 53 | 69 | 2500 | 2.0 | Tremor ++ Dizziness ++ Vomiting ++ Diarrhea ++ | 527 | 65 | 100 | Dizziness | 1500 | 1.4 |
| 508 | 50 | 138 | 2000 | 1.7 | Asymptomatic | | | | | | |
| 511 | 55 | 53 | 2000 | 2.45 | Tremor Weight loss Toxic confusion* | | | | | | |

*Treatment was discontinued.

obviously demonstrated by the Efficacity Index (EI)*. Although the EI was 1.86 for the whole lithium group, it was only 1.72 with the original dosage and 2.08 for the revised dosage.

## 8.   Importance of the Placebo Group

While in the total Hamilton score, lithium and clomipramine both proved to be significantly more potent than placebo, this did not appear in the Clinical Global Impression, where only lithium was significantly better than placebo with p <0.05. There was also a significant improvement in the placebo group between the initial and final weeks according to the total Hamilton score. Possibly, this derives in part from the significant improvement noted in Factor I (sleep disturbances), as a result of the use of hypnotic drugs. Nevertheless, this particular improvement with placebo should be stressed, as well as the fact that five additional patients who had been admitted to this study improved and hence dropped out during the washing-out period with placebo. We would like to mention here that Klein and Davis (1969) found in their review that of 11 out of 36 controlled studies comparing imipramine to placebo, there was no significant difference between the 2 medications. Honigfeld (1968) already pointed out the various nonspecific factors improving the condition of hospitalized, depressed patients, in particular those participating in a psychopharmacological trial. Such are the milieu, the investigator's enthusiasm, and the patients' confidence in the treatment. The importance of a placebo group as additional control is therefore unquestionable to us.

## E.   FURTHER CLINICAL PROBLEMS

## 1.   The Use of Lithium in Severe Depressive States

The results of our study, comparing lithium to a known antidepressant drug, were similar to those reported by Mendels et al. (1972) and Watanabe et al. (1975): Lithium is an antidepressant agent at least as effective as known tricyclic antidepressants such as imipramine and clomipramine. Lithium also proved to be effective in severe depressive states, provided that it is used in appropriate dosage. For that matter, our conclusions were identical to those of Mendels et al. (1972) who like ourselves, treated severe depressive patients and reached doses similar to the ones we used, but differed from the opinions of Fieve et al. (1968) and Watanabe et al. (1975), who both warned against the use of lithium in severe depression.

---

*The Efficacity Index is measured by the ratio between the therapeutic effect and the side effects.

## 2.  Time-Lapse Changes With Lithium

When does lithium start to show its effect upon severely depressed patients? It is generally accepted that, in manic states, the full effect of lithium appears between the sixth and the tenth day with an adequate dosage of the drug (Gershon, 1970; Arieli, 1972; Peet, 1975).

In depressive states, the antidepressant effect of lithium seems more delayed. Nahuneck et al. (1970) claimed that 54 percent of endogenous-depressive patients responded, as did the manic patients, between the end of the first week and the beginning of the second week of treatment, but theirs was an uncontrolled ial using a wide range of doses (300 to 2,000 mg) during varying periods of time. Watanabe et al. (1975) reported that the action of lithium appeared at the end of the first week and so preceded the effect of imipramine, but there was no significant difference in rapidity of action between the two drugs. Mendels et al. (1972) found no difference in latency for the therapeutic effect of lithium versus desimipramine: There was a progressive weekly improvement that reached a maximum at the end of the third week.

Like Mendels and his co-workers, we found no significant difference in rapidity of action between lithium and clomipramine. In both cases, some improvement appeared at the end of the first week, but a significant response was only obtained at the end of the second week of treatment. At that time, the effect of clomipramine seemed to be somewhat stronger (Figure 1). There was some further development: Although lithium still showed a significant effect on depressed patients who had not responded before, it seemed that clomipramine had shown most of its action by the end of the second week. Therefore we drew the following conclusions:
1. There seems to be no relevant difference in latency of action between lithium and clomipramine.
2. Lithium is similar, for that matter, to all the known groups of antidepressants, i.e., secondary and tertiary tricyclics and MAOI, for which the main effect appears at the end of the second week. This latency is an interesting psychopharmacological phenomenon that has not yet been satisfactorily explained.
3. It is not logical to discontinue treatment with an adequate dosage of lithium in patients who show no improvement after 2 weeks. It is worthwhile to proceed for at least another week.

## 3.  Adequate Dosage of Lithium in Treatment of Acute Depression

The problem of adequate dosage of lithium is crucial in acute depressive states. An excessive dosage might induce severe neurotoxic symptoms, as occurred in the first part of our study. On the other hand, too low a dosage might fail to show an antidepressant effect, and results will not be reliable, as occurred in several studies mentioned above.

In our trial, the average, adequate therapeutic dosage of lithium carbonate was considered to be about double the necessary prophylactic dosage, i.e., 1,500 to 2,000 mg per day. These doses are comparable for their effect to 150 to 200 mg of clomipramine. Such dosage appears to be effective in treating severe depressive states. We reached this conclusion after long experience in our outpatient clinic for prophylactic treatment as well as treatment of hospitalized patients. Mendels et al. (1972) used a similar doses and obtained comparable results. Increasing the dosage above 2,500 mg per day proved unwiser, as it did not bring further improvement, but induced neurotoxic reactions. Our opinion thus differs from Neubauer et al. (1976), who found it necessary to reach a toxic effect in about half of their patients in order to achieve improvement. Naturally, the maximal dosage should be reached progressively and prudently in order to avoid initial concomitant symptoms, such as gastrointestinal disorders and severe tremor, which could prevent the patient from reaching an adequate dosage of lithium.

One must also consider the patient's weight and age. With elderly patients, it is advisable not to give more than 1,500 mg per day, since their tolerance to lithium seems somewhat reduced. This might be partially related to the fact that low values of lithium clearance (10 ml/min instead of about 20 ml/min), as well as of creatinine clearance, have been reported in elderly patients by Schou (1969). Although Fyrö et al. (1973) does not confirm this finding in his series, we suspect that such a reduction does occur, especially since the risk of impaired renal function is greater in older patients.

Furthermore, the lithium clearance diminishes when sodium intake and sodium clearance, are reduced, since there is competition between lithium and sodium for active transport mechanism in the proximal tubes of the nephron. A proper diet and fluid intake should also be insured for the above reasons and because of the tendency of depressed patients to reduce their food and fluid intake. In such cases, reducing and dividing the daily maximal dosage is preferred. Furthermore, serum lithium levels should be measured once or twice a week and should be prevented from varying too much from the 1.0 mEq/liter level. When possible, it is recommended to determine the red blood cell (RBC) to plasma lithium ratio (Elizur et al., 1975), as will be discussed below. All the above and the difficulty, in our experience, to adequately supervise drug treatment in ambulatory patients, leads us to prefer hospitalization when lithium is to be used effectively as an antidepressant.

4.  Types of Depression, Biochemical Features, and Predictability of Response to Treatment

a.  Unipolar Versus Bipolar Depression

Of all the classifications of depression, the subdivision into unipolar and bipolar categories aroused the most interest as far as lithium treatment is concerned. The first studies of Fieve et al. (1968), Dyson and Mendels (1968), and Goodwin et al. (1972) stressed the fact that lithium is particularly effective in bipolar-depressive patients. Later controlled studies failed to confirm these findings. Mendels (1976) and Watanabe et al. (1975) did not report a significantly better effect of lithium on bipolar patients. In our research, as mentioned before, a greater improvement was found in the bipolar group as compared with the unipolar one. But in our study, as well as in others, in which the effect of lithium was studied comparatively in the two diagnostic subgroups, the number of patients was too small to allow a proper statistical evaluation. On the other hand, the experience of the last few years has somewhat lessened the initial enthusiasm for this subdivision, which was first proposed by Kraepelin (1904), and reawakened interest in the 1960s when Perris (1966) and Winokur and Cleyton (1967) described differences in family history of the patients and concluded that there were genetic differences between the two subgroups.

Indeed, from a clinical point of view, Mendels (1976) correctly observed that typical unipolar patients might, later in their lives, also suffer manic episodes. Baron et al. (1975) found neither genetically determined changes in red blood cell catechol-o-methyl-transferase (COMT) nor differences in the Visual Average Evoked Response (AER) between bipolar and unipolar patients. Thus they contradict the previous findings of Buchsbaum et al. (1971) who described changes in AER in these two groups.

### b. Other Biochemical Features

Serry (1969) claimed that response to lithium could be predicted by the urinary secretion of lithium in a 4-hour period after ingestion of a single oral dose of 1,200 mg of lithium, but his findings could not be confirmed.

Of greater importance is the determination of the RBC lithium/plasma lithium ratio (LR), as depressed patients who respond to lithium have been found to have a consistently higher lithium ratio than non-lithium responders. This difference appears independent of the dose of lithium and of the plasma-lithium concentration. As the LR tends to stabilize early in the course of treatment, a high level of this ratio can be used as a predictor of clinical improvements (Mendels and Frazer 1973). These authors also reported that male control subjects had a relatively lower LR than their lithium responders (mainly manic-depressive); while female manic depressives, according to Lyttkens et al. (1973) had a significantly higher LR than controlled subjects. On the contrary, Elizur et al. (1972, 1978) found the LR of patients in acute polar phase of manic-depressive illness to be lower than in their normothymic phase and lower than in healthy individuals. Nor did they find in their sample a significant difference in LR between responders in manic phase, as well as in depressive phase, and non-responders.

On the other hand, Elizur et al. (1972, 1975), emphasized the value of a high LR as a sensitive indicator for impending neurotoxicity, even in patients with serum lithium levels still within therapeutic range. A critical value of 60 percent for the lithium ratio was described.

Mendels (1976) also examined the RBC sodium concentrations during lithium treatment in depressed patients and found that patients who showed an increase in this factor were more likely to improve and that the LR was significantly higher in lithium-treated patients whose base-line sodium concentration was higher.

A relatively high base-line calcium-magnesium ratio in plasma, and an initial increase in plasma magnesium and calcium have also been reported to correlate with a positive antidepressant response to lithium (Carman et al., 1974).

Urinary 3-methoxy-4-hydroxyphenylglycol (MHPG) excretion, considered to reflect norepinephrine (NE) metabolism in the brain, is also of importance, as it was reported to be lower in bipolar depressive patients than in patients with unipolar disorders and than in normal controls; it was also reported to increase after recovery and to be high in the manic phase. Maas (1975) identified two subgroups of depressive patients. Those who had a low pretreatment level of 24-hour urinary excretion of MHPG showed a positive response to imipramine and norimipramine; they reacted by a brightening of mood when administered amphetamine, and did not respond to amitriptyline. The other subgroup of patients who showed a normal or high pretreatment level of urinary MHPG did not react to either imipramine, norimipramine, or amphetamine, but responded to amitriptyline. Schildkraut (1973), treating a heterogenous group of depressive patients also obtained a "rapid and sustained response" to amitriptyline in patients with a higher pretreatment level of MHPG and other NE metabolites, while those with a low level did not respond as such. Interestingly, the patients with the lowest levels of MHPG and other NE metabolites were bipolar.

On the other hand, there is pharmacological evidence from studies in animals that the various tricyclic antidepressants (TCA) have different effects on the uptake of the various amines. Thus, secondary amine TCA would have a preferential effect on NE re-uptake, while the tertiary amine derivatives would act through the serotonine system. Imipramine, a tertiary amine, being rapidly metabolized in the liver into desimipramine, acts in vivo mainly as a secondary amine. Clomipramine, for its part, maintains its principal activity as a tertiary amine.

MHPG may thus provide a biochemical criterion for differential responses to treatment with tricyclic antidepressants. It is still difficult to fit lithium into this scheme, as its action upon the amine transmitters seems rather the opposite of that which is considered to be a possible mechanism of action of the TCA. Nevertheless, bipolar depression has been reported to represent a "clinically identifiable subgroup" of the depressive disorders characterized biochemically by a relatively low MHPG excretion (Schild-kraut 1978).

Finally, attention was attracted to the fact that lithium responders were found to have a significantly lower pretreatment level of platelet MAO than non-responders, without any overlap in values between the two groups (Wilson et al., 1975).

### c. Agitated Versus Retarded Depression

The differential effect of antidepressant drugs upon agitated or retarded depressions aroused the interest of clinicians in the 1970s. Bielski and Friedel (1976), in their exhaustive review of numerous studies, compared the effects of imipramine and amitriptyline. They concluded that imipramine was effective only in depression with psychomotor retardation, whereas ami-triptyline was also active in psychomotor agitation. Hippius (1972) con-firmed that amitriptyline had a positive effect in agitated depression, while the imipramine derivatives (such as imipramine, clomipramine, and desimipramine) showed a depression-relieving and a psychomotor activating action rather than a sedative one.

Roth et al. (1976) claimed that only MAOI antidepressants had a sedative effect in agitated depression. On the contrary, Hynes (1973) reported a sedative effect for clomipramine similar to amitriptyline and a positive effect on the factors of agitation and anxiety in depression. His study refers to outpatients only.

As far as lithium is concerned, few studies were reported that dealt with its differential effect on the two important factors discussed here. Nahuneck et al. (1970) found lithium to be less effective in retarded depression than desimipramine or noramitriptyline (which are both demethylated tricyclic antidepressants), but it proved superior in anxious and agitated depressive states. It should be stressed again, however, that this was an open trial. On the other hand, Watanabe et al. (1975), in a controlled study with imipra-mine, found that the component of anxiety and agitation was significantly more influenced by imipramine than by lithium.

In our study, we confirmed the findings of Nahuneck et al. (1970), concerning the positive effect of lithium in anxious and agitated depression, which is contradictory to the conclusions of Watanabe et al. (1975). We found lithium to be more effective than clomipramine for sedation of agitated depression, although not significantly so. Clomipramine on the other hand, proved superior in retarded depressive states. It is possible that this contradiction to Watanabe et al. stems from the smaller dosage that they used and the higher scores for anxiety reported for our patients. We also have to consider the relatively older age of our patients, an average of 50.07 years: They naturally fit in the age group of "involutional depression," which is often characterized by an agitated depressive state. Lithium would thus be indicated in this group age as also amitriptyline and MAOI. Here again, we should stress the difference between the two subgroups of tricyclic antidepressants. The secondary amines, acting mainly through the noradrenergic system, are reported to be more activating; while the tertiary amines, which act mainly through the serotonine system, are more sedative.

### d. A Special Syndrome

Neubauer and Bermingham (1976) recently described a depressive syndrome characterized by obsessive features responding to lithium (see Table 4). They cited Gittleson (1966), who observed that about one third of depressed patients complain of obsessive symptoms. In our study, 18 of the 33 patients showed mild obsessive symptoms. Lithium had indeed a better effect than the two other medications tested upon these symptoms.

### 5. Lithium in Combination with Other Antidepressants

Several studies, most of them uncontrolled, emphasize the potentiation by lithium of other antidepressant drugs. Zall et al. (1968) used lithium to potentiate the effect of isocarboxazide, an antidepressant of the MAOI group. Himmelhoch et al. (1972) similarly described the potentiation of another I, tranylcypromine. More recently, Neubauer and Bermingham (1976) reported that depressed patients with obsessive symptoms, who had not reacted either to antidepressant medication or to electroconvulsive therapy (ECT), responded positively to the combined use of lithium and tranylcypramine.

Lingjaerde et al. (1974) were the only investigators to conduct a controlled study on the subject. They found the concomitant use of lithium and tricyclic antidepressant superior to the latter only.

Table 4.  Effect on Obsessive Symptoms in Hamilton Scale

|  | Lithium | | Clomipramine | | Placebo | |
|---|---|---|---|---|---|---|
|  | No. | Percent | No. | Percent | No. | Percent |
| Total | 5 | 100 | 6 | 100 | 7 | 100 |
| Improvement | 4 | 80 | 3 | 50 | 2 | 28.5 |
| No Improvement | 1 | 20 | 3 | 50 | 5 | 71.5 |

## ACKNOWLEDGEMENTS

The authors wish to thank Professor S. Gershon, with whom this study was planned during Dr. A. Arieli's research fellowship at the Psychopharmacology Research Unit, N.Y.U. Medical Center. The authors are grateful to Dr. Guy and his associates of the Biometric Laboratory of the NIMH and to Ms. Rivka Reznik of the Statistics Department of Kupath Holim, who were both very helpful in the statistical assessment of our results.

This study was supported by grants from the Office of the Chief Scientist, Israel Health Ministry, and from the Israeli Center for Psychobiology.

# F. REFERENCES

American Psychiatric Association (1968). Diagnostic and Statistical Manual of Mental Disorders. 2nd edition. Am. Psychiat. Ass., Washington, D.C.

Andreani, G., Caselli, G., and Martelli, G. (1958). Ritievi clinici ed. electtro encefalografici durante il trattemento con sali di lito in malati psichiatrici. G. Psichiat. Neuropatol. 86:273-328.

Arieli, A. (1972). Lithium carbonate in acute manic reaction. Harefuah. 182:235-259.

Baron, M., Gershon, E.S., Rudy, V. et al. (1975). Lithium carbonate response in depression. Prediction by unipolar/bipolar illness, average-evoked response, catechol-O-methyltransferase, and family history. Arch. Gen. Psychiat. 32:9:1107-1111.

Beck, A.T., Ward, C., Mendelson, M., Mock, J., and Ejbaugh J. (1961). An inventory for measuring depression. Arch. Gen. Psychiat. 4:561-571.

Bennie, E.H. (1975). (Letter) Lithium in depression. Lancet. 1:216.

Bielski, R.J., and Friedel, R.O. (1976). Prediction of tricyclic antidepressant response: A critical review. Arch. Gen. Psychiat. 33:1479-1489.

Buchsbaum, M., Goodwin, F.K., Murphy, D.L., (1971). Average revoked responses in affective disorders. Am. J. Psychiat. 128:19-25.

Cade, J.G.J. (1949). Lithium salts in the treatment of psychiatric excitement. Med. J. Aust. 36:349-352.

Carman, J.S., Post, R.M., Teplitz, T.A., and Goodwin, F.K. (1974). (Letter) Divalent cations in predicting antidepressant responde to lithium. Lancet. 2:1454.

Clinical Global Impression (CGI) ECDEU Assessment Manual for Psychopharmacology, revised. (1976). W. Guy, ed. U.S. Department of Health, Education, and Welfare, Washington D.C.

Dyson, W.L., and Mendels, J. (1968). Lithium and depression. Curr. Ther. Res. 10:601-608.

Elizur, A., Graff, E., Segal, Z., Yeret, A., and Davidson, S. (1978). Red blood cell./plasma ratio in acute effective state during the course of lithium therapy. (In press.)

Elizur, A., Graff, E., Steiner, M., and Davidson, S. (1977). Acute lithium toxicity and its physiological correlates. Harefuah. 92:248-251.

Elizur A., Graff, E., Steiner, M., and Davidson, S. (1975). Intra/extra red blood cell lithium and electrolyte distributions as correlates of neurotoxic reactions during lithium therapy, in The Impact of Biology of Modern Psychiatry. E.S. Gershon, ed. Plenum Press, New York and London.

Elizur, A., Shopsin, B., Gershon, S., and Ehlenberger, A. (1972). Intra/extracellular lithium ratios and clinical course in affective states. Clin. Pharmacol. Therapeut. 13:947-952.

Fieve, R.R., Platman, S.R., and Plutchik, R.R. (1968). The use of lithium in affective disorders. I. Acute endogenous depression. Am J. Psychiat. 125:487-491.

Fyrö, B., Petterson, U., and Sedvall, G. (1973). Pharmacokinetics of lithium in manic-depressive patients. Acta Psychiat. Scand. 49:237-247.

Gershon, S., (1970). Lithium in mania. *Clin. Pharmacol. Therapy.* 11:168-187.

Gittleson, N.L., (1966). Depressive psychosis in the obsessional neurotic. *Brit. J. Psychiatry* 112:883-887.

Goodwin, F.K., Murphy, D.L., and Bunney, W.E., Jr. (1969). Lithium-carbonate treatment in depression and mania. A longitudinal double-blind study. *Arch. Gen. Psychiat.* 21:486-496.

Goodwin, F.K., Murphy, D.L., Dunner, D.L., and Bunney, W.G., Jr. (1972). Lithium response in unipolar versus bipolar depression. *Am. J. Psychiat.* 129:44-47.

Hamilton, M. (1967). Development of a rating scale for primary affective illness. *Brit. J. Soc. Clin. Psychol.* 6:278-296.

Hamilton, M. (1960). A rating scale for depression. *J. Neurol. Neurosurg. Psychiat.* 23:56-62.

Hansen, C.J., Retboll, K., and Schou, M., (Unpublished study quoted by Schou, 1968.)

Himmelhoch, J.M., Detre, T., Kupfer, D.J., Swartzburg, M., and Byck, R. (1972). Treatment of previously intractable depressions with tranylcypromine and lithium. *J. Nerv. Ment. Dis.* 155:216-220.

Hippius, H. (1972). The current status of treatment for depression, in *Depressive Illness, Diagnosis, Assessment, Treatment.* P. Kielholz ed. Hans Huber Publishers, Bern. pp. 49-56.

Honigfeld, G. (1968). Specific and non-specific factors in the treatment of depressed states, in *Non-Specific Factors in Drug Therapy.* K. Rickels, ed. Charles C. Thomas, Springfield. pp. 80-107.

Hynes, M.V. (1973). A comparative clinical trial of oral clomipramine (Anafranil) against amitriptyline. *J. Int. Med. Res.* 1:338-342.

Johnson, G. (1974). Antidepressant effect of lithium. *Comp. Psychiat.* 15:43-47.

Klein, D.F., and Davis, J.M. (1969). *Diagnosis and Drug Treatment of Psychiatric Disorders.* Williams & Wilkins, Baltimore.

Kraepelin, E. (1904). *Lecture on Clinical Psychiatry.* Builliere, Tindall, and Cox, London.

Lingjaerde, O., Edlund, A.H., Gormsen, C.A., Gottfries, C.G., Haugstad, A., Hermann, I.L., Hollnagel, P., Mäkimattilla, A., Rassmussen, K.E., Remvig, J., and Robak, O.H. (1974). The effects of lithium-carbonate in combination with tricyclic antidepressants in endogenous depression. A double-blind, multicenter trial. *Acta Psychiat. Scand.* 50:233-242.

Lyttkens, L., Söderberg, U., and Wetterberg, L. (1973). Increased lithium erythrocyte plasma ratio in manic-depressive psychosis. *Lancet.* 1:40.

Maas, J.W. (1975). Biogenic amines and depression: Biochemical and pharmacological separation of two types of depression. *Arch. Gen. Psychi.* 32:1357-1361.

Mendels, J. (1976). Lithium in the treatment of depression. *Am. J. Psychiat.* 133:373-378.

Mendels, J. (1975). Lithium in the acute treatment of depressive states, in *Lithium Research and Therapy.* F.N. Johnson, ed. Academic Press, New York. pp. 43-62.

Mendels, J., and Frazer, A. (1973). Intracellular lithium concentration and clinical response: Towards a membrane theory of depression. *J. Psychiat. Res.* 10:9-18.

Mendels, J., Secunda, S.K., and Dyson, W.L. (1972). A controlled study of the antidepressant effects of lithium. *Arch. Gen. Psychiat.* 26:154-157.

Nahuneck, K., Svestka, J., and Rodová, A. (1970). Zur Stellung des Lithiums in der Gruppe der Antidepressiva in der Behandlung von akuten endogenen und Involutions-Depréssionen. (The position of lithium among antidepressants in the treatment of acute phases of endogenous and involutional depressions.) *Int. Pharmaco-Psychiat.* 5:249-257.

Neubauer H. and Bermingham, P. (1976). A depressive syndrome responsive to lithium. An analysis of 20 cases. *J. Nerv. Ment. Dis.* 163:4:276-281.

Noack, C.H., and Trautner, E.M. (1951). The lithium treatment of maniacal psychosis. *Med. J. Aust.* 38:219-222.

Noyes, R., Jr., Dempsey, G.M., Blum, A., and Cavanaugh, G.L. (1974). Lithium treatment of depression. *Comp. Psychiat.* 15:187-193.

Noyes, R., Jr., Ringdahl, J.C., and Andreasen, N.J. (1971). Effect of lithium citrate on adrenocortical activity in manic depressive illness. *Comp. Psychiat.* 12:337-347.

Peet, M. (1975). Lithium in the acute treatment of mania, in *Lithium Research and Therapy.* F.N. Johnson, ed. Academic Press, New York. pp. 25-41.

Perris, C.A. (1966). A study of bipolar (manic-depressive) and unipolar recurrent depressive psychosis. *Acta Psychiat. Scand.* (Supp. 194) 42:1-199.

Roth, M., Gurney, C., Mountjoy, C.Q., Kerr, T.A., and Schapira, K. (1976). The relationship between classification and response to drugs in affective disorders—problems posed by drug response in affective disorders, in *Monamine Oxidase and its Inhibition.* Ciba Foundation Symposium, 39 (New Series), Elsevier, Excerpta Medica, North Holland. Amsterdam, Oxford, New York. pp. 297-319.

Schildkraut, J.J. (1978). The biochemistry of affective disorders: A brief summary, in *Harvard Guide to Modern Psychiatry.* A.M. Nicholi, ed. The Belknap Press of Harvard University Press. Cambridge, pp. 81-91.

Schildkraut, J.J. (1973). Norepinephrine metabolites as biochemical criteria for classifying depressive disorders and predicting responses to treatment: Preliminary findings. *Am. J. Psychiat.* 130:695-699.

Schou, M. (1969). Lithium: Relation between clinical effects of the drug and its absorption, distribution, and excretion, in *The Present Status of Psychotropic Drugs.* A Cerletti and F.S. Bove, eds. Exerpta Medica Foundation, Amsterdam. pp. 120-122.

Schou, M. (1968). Lithium in psychiatric therapy and prophylaxis. *J. Psychiat. Res.* 5:67-95.

Serry, M. (1969). The lithium excretion test. *Aust. N.Z.L. Psychiat.* 3:390-392.

Spitzer, R.L., Endicott, J., and Fleiss, J.L. (1967). Instrument and recording forms for evaluating psychiatric status and history: Rationale, method, and description. *Comp. Psychiat.* 8:321-343.

Stokes, P.E., Shamoian, C.A., Stoll, P.M., and Patton, M.J. (1971). Efficacy of lithium as acute treatment of manic-depressive illness. *Lancet.* 1:1319-1325.

Van der Velde, C.D. (1970). Effectiveness of lithium-carbonate in the treatment of manic-depressive illness. *Am. J. Psychiat.* 127:345-351.

Vojtechovsky, M. (1957). Zkusenosti s lecbou solemi lithia, in *Problemy Psychiatrie v Praxi a ve Vyskumu.* (quoted by Schou, 1968).

Watanabe, S., Ishino H., and Otsuki, S. (1975). Double-blind comparison of lithium-carbonate and imipramine in treatment of depression. *Arch. Gen. Psychiat.* 32:659-668.

Wilson, S., Dyson, W., and Mendels, J. (1975). In preparation, quoted by Mendels (1975). Lithium in the acute treatment of depressive states, in *Lithium Research and Therapy,* F.N. Johnson, ed. Academic Press, New York. p. 62.

Winokur, C., and Cleyton, P.J. (1967). Family history studies: I. Two types of affective disorders separated according to genetic and clinical factors, in *Recent Advances in Biological Psychiatry,* Volume 9. I.J. Works, ed. Plenum Press, New York. pp. 35-50.

Worrall, E.P., Moody, J.P., Peet, M., Dick, P., Smith, A., Chambers, C., Adams, M., and Naylor, G.J. (1979). Controlled studies of the acute antidepressant effects of lithium. *Brit. J. Psychiat.* 135:255-262.

Zall, H., Therman, P.O.G., and Myers, J.M. (1968). Lithium carbonate: A clinical study. *Am. J. Psychiat.* 125:549-555.

Zuckermann, M. (1960). The development of an affect adjective check list for the measurement of anxiety. *J. Consult. Psychol.* 24:457-462.

Current Developments in Psychopharmacology, Volume 6
© 1981, Spectrum Publications, Inc.

CHAPTER 7

# CHRONOPHARMACOLOGICAL STUDIES OF NEUROLEPTICS

HARUO NAGAYAMA
AKINORI TAKAGI
RYO TAKAHASHI

Studies were carried out to clarify the mechanism of appearance and the laws controlling the appearance of such phenomena as circadian fluctuation in the effects of neuroleptics. A detailed review was initially made of previous studies on drugs closely related to neuroleptics; then data obtained by the authors was analyzed. Significant circadian fluctuation was found in the effect of chlorpromazine, haloperidol, and tetrabenazine, varying with the time of administration, with the kind of drug, and even with the dose of the same drug. There was also circadian fluctuation in lethality rate, which was seen to be a phenomenon controlled by a law different from that controlling circadian fluctuation in the effect of a drug. Circadian fluctuation in the effect of a drug was regulated externally by clock time, setting the light-dark rhythm of the raising environment. Different times of administration of a drug did not affect chronological changes in the blood level or intracerebral concentration of a drug after administration. From these results, it was assumed that this phenomenon might be induced by the circadian rhythm of drug sensitivity of the brain where the drug acts.

## A. INTRODUCTION

It has been conventionally accepted that when the same dose of a drug is administered to a given living organism, the drug will always exert the same action upon the organism and give rise to the same response, regardless of the time of administration. This concept, however, is too simple, since the living organism is continuously displaying various types of circadian rhythm (biological rhythm, having a period of about 24 hours). It can be assumed that the response of the organism to a drug may also fluctuate in concomitance with these biological fluctuations. Many drugs have been examined on the basis of this assumption. As a result, it has been shown that there is a circadian fluctuation in the effects of these drugs, and that the amplitude of effect of the same drug can change greatly if the time of drug administration (TODA) is changed. These observations are taken out of the laboratory and applied to clinical practice (Moore Ede, 1973; Reinberg, 1973).

As far as neuroleptics are concerned, studies have just been initiated on the above-mentioned subject. The clarification of this subject may lead to a better understanding of the mechanism of action of these drugs and of the function of the brain. Moreover, it may also bring about the development of a new method of treatment, including the determination of single daily doses of a drug in clinical practice. Therefore, this problem should be resolved as early as possible. The present paper deals with the circadian fluctuation in the effect of neuroleptics, or in the susceptibility of the living organism to these drugs.

There are at least three main issues in the study on the relationship between drugs and biological rhythms:

1. The toxicity of a drug varying with TODA, or the fluctuation of lethality rate due to the difference in TODA (circadian chronotoxicology).
2. The fluctuation of the drug effects, depending on TODA.
3. The drug influence upon the various rhythms of living organisms.

The third issue seems to be somewhat out of place in the present investigation. Consequently, this chapter will deal exclusively with the first two issues.

## B. FLUCTUATION OF PSYCHOTROPIC DRUG TOXICITY, ACCORDING TO THE DIFFERENCE IN TODA

Various experiments to study the lethality rate have been conducted in animals raised in environments where conditions of illumination and temperature were strictly controlled. The drugs used were pentobarbital, phenobarbital, ethanol, amphetamine, chlordiazepoxide, chlorpromazine, and lithium. All the drugs tested showed a significant circadian fluctuation of their lethality rate. The results of these experiments are summarized in Table 1. In each experiment, the daytime was divided into 12-hour light and dark periods, and the actual clock hour was converted to the time after the beginning of the light period.

A review of Table 1 reveals that there are considerable differences reported by the previous investigators in the time of appearance of a crest, even when the same drug was administered; for example, there is a difference as great as 12 hours in the data reported on the administration of chlorpromazine by Hata et al. (1975) and by Nagayama et al. (1978c). However, it is presumed that such differences may disappear with the use of a more precise method, which would eliminate, for example, differences in the animal species used. In addition, it is important to note that when the experimental method of the two groups was compared, there was a difference in length of the preadministration period used to adopt the experimental animals to the light-dark rhythm of raising environments. This period was more than 1 week in the experiment carried out by Hata et al., and more than 5 weeks in that by Nagayama et al.

It should be noted that the time period in Hata's experiment was extremely short. The administration dose also differed: 250 mg/kg in the experiment by Hata et al., and 74 mg/kg in the experiment by Nagayama et al. It is noted that the dose was extremely large in the experiment by Hata et al. In all the experimental groups except one, in the experiment by Hata et al., more than 90 percent of the animals died within 72 hours. Therefore, the lethality rate fluctuated within a narrow range of 90 to 100 percent, and the difference in time was indistinct. In this case, the velocity of occurrence of death was regarded as an important factor, rather than the final lethality rate. In the experiement performed by Nagayama et al., the dose conventionally regarded as $LD_{50}$ was administered. Accordingly, the lethality rate reached a high of 75.0 percent at the end of an observation period of 13 days. Since it fluctuated in a wide range from 33.3 to 75.0 percent, this clearly indicates the difference in toxicity of a drug between any two times of its administration.

In conventional pharmacological research, a method has been extensively applied in which $LD_{50}$ is used as one of the indicators of the intensity of toxicity of a drug. As mentioned above, there is a circadian fluctuation in lethality rate, and the ratio of fluctuation has even reached 11.7 in a certain drug. It seems necessary to adopt the concept of time for the determination of $LD_{50}$; therefore, $LD_{50}$ may be indicated for a given time as $LD_{50}/TODA$. If this method is too complicated, it is possible to replace it by a method in which $LD_{50}$ is determined for the time when the toxicity of the drug is expressed to the largest extent.

Scheving (1968) reported that when amphetamine was administered, a rat made blind by bilateral enucleation still presented a rhythm in spite of the occurrence of a phase shift; he suggested that the light-dark rhythm of the environment might have acted as a synchronizer. Nelson and Halberg

**Table 1. Circadian Fluctuation of Lethality Rate Caused by Various Psychotropic Drugs Administered at Different Times** *

| Drugs | Doses (i.p.) | Species and Sex | Time Showing Highest Lethality Rate | | Ratio of Crest to Trough | Remarks | References |
|---|---|---|---|---|---|---|---|
| | | | Light Period | Dark Period | | | |
| Pentobarbital | 75 mg/kg | S.D. rat | | ↑ | 2.6 | | Pauly and Schevinger, 1964 |
| | 85 mg/kg | S.D. rat | | ↑ | 5.0 | | |
| | 90 mg/kg | S.D. rat | | ← | 3.0 | | |
| | 130 mg/kg | Swiss mouse (F) | Experiment was carried out only during the light period | | — | | Lindsay and Kullman, 1966 |
| Phenobarbital | — | Swiss–Webster mouse (M) | ⌐← | | 1.1 | Calculation of LD$_{50}$ | Walker and Owasoyo, 1974 |
| Ethanol | 0.2 ml | C-mouse (M) | | ← | 7.0 | | Haus and Halberg, 1959 |
| | 6 mg/kg | BALB/c mouse (M&F) | | ← | — | | Nelson and Halberg, 1973 |
| D-amphetamine | 26–30 mg/kg | S.D. rat (M) | | ↑ | 11.7 | | Scheving, 1968, 1969 |
| Dl-amphetamine | — | Mouse | | ⌐↑ | 1.2† / 1.9 | Calculation of LD$_{50}$ | Walker, 1974 |
| Chlordiazepoxide | — | D$_8$ and B$_1$ mouse | ← | | — | | Marte and Halberg, 1961 |

**Time Showing Highest Lethality Rate**

| Drugs | Doses (i.p.) | Species and Sex | Light Period | Dark Period | Ratio of Crest to Trough | Remarks | References |
|---|---|---|---|---|---|---|---|
| Chlorpromazine | 74 mg/kg | S.D. rat (M) | | | ↑ 2.2 | | Nagayama et al., 1978c |
| | 250 mg/kg | dd mouse (M) | | ↑ | | | Hata et al., 1975 |
| Lithium | 940 mg/kg | Swiss–Webster mouse (M) | ↑ | | — | | Hawkins et al., 1978 |

* All the agents were used in an experiment with a 12-hour light and 12-hour dark period in a day. In this table, all the times are expressed as relative clock times counted from the beginning of the light.
† The upper level indicates results from isolated mice, and the lower level results from aggregated mice.

(1973b) pointed out that when ethanol was administered and when the light-dark rhythm was so controlled as to be 12 hours earlier or later than the accustomed one, a phase shift occurred accordingly in the rhythm of lethality rate. Nelson et al. therefore draws the same conclusions from their experiment as Scheving.

## C. FLUCTUATION IN EFFECT OF PSYCHOTROPIC DRUGS DUE TO DIFFERENCE IN TODA

As Shown in Table 2, a circadian fluctuation has been demonstrated in the effects of pentobarbital, hexobarbital, phenobarbital, ethanol, p-chlormethamphetamine, methamphetamine, d-amphetamine, tetrabenazine, chlorpromazine, and haloperiodol. Furthermore, Davies et al. (1973) reported results obtained from amphetamine, LSD, and mescaline. They discussed the absolute value of each indicator (the number of entries into the arm of the Y-maze and rear) when a drug had been administered, but failed to present the ratio of change of the drug administration group against the untreated control group. Therefore, the paper of Davies et al. was not evaluated in the present study, since it could not be discussed from the point of view of this paper.

In this section the drugs mentioned above are discussed, with the exception of neuroleptics. An outstanding fact of Table 2 is that in the case of the first five drugs listed—the barbiturates, ethanol, and p-chlormethamphetamine—almost all the data had a crest in the light period; but only in the case of methamphetamine and d-amphetamine, a crest was found in the dark period. From these results, it seems that, with a few exceptions, inhibitory drugs may exhibit a crest in the light period (non-active stage), and stimulative drugs may show a crest in the dark period (active stage).

Actually, however, the relationship between the character of a drug and the appearance of a crest is not so simple. Even when the same drug was administered, the time of appearance of a crest varied with the dose administered. For example, in the case of pentobarbital, when a small dose was administered, a crest appeared at the end of the light period or in the transitional stage from the light to the dark period. When there was an increase in the dose of administration, the crest was shifted to the left-hand side of Table 2, or the beginning of the light period, regardless of the difference between investigators, or between the species of experimental animals. As mentioned below, this phenomenon also appeared when neuroleptics were administered, although in a different form. Therefore, it cannot be regarded as an incidental phenomenon. It will be discussed further in the following section.

## Table 2. Circadian Fluctuation of Effectiveness Caused by Various Psychotropic Drugs Administered at Different Times

| Drugs | Doses (mg/kg) (i.p.) | Species and Sex | Time of Administration When Maximum Response was Shown to Drug (Light Period / Dark Period) | Ratio of Crest to Trough | Variables Investigated | References |
|---|---|---|---|---|---|---|
| Pentobarbital | 35 | S.D. rat (M) | ↑ Dark Period | 1.7 | Duration of anesthesia | Scheving et al., 1968b |
| | 50 | S.D. rat (M) | ↑ Light Period | 1.4 | Onset of sleep (minimum) | Friedman et al., 1969 |
| | 50 | S.D. rat (M) | ↑ Light Period | 1.9 | Duration of sleep | |
| | 60 | Swiss mouse (M) | ↑ Light Period | 1.8 | Duration of sleep | Davis, 1962 |
| | 65 | BALB/cCr mouse (M) | ↑ Light Period | – | Duration of anesthesia | Nelson and Halberg, 1973a |
| | 71.5 | BALB/cCr mouse (M) | ↑ Light Period | – | Duration of sleep | |
| | 78.7 | BALB/cCr mouse (M) | ↑ Light Period | – | Duration of sleep | |
| | 86.5 | BALB/cCr mouse (M) | ↑ Light Period | – | Duration of sleep | |
| | 100 | Deer mouse | 10 to 20% more rapid during the dark phase than during the light phase | – | Rate of recovery from anesthesia | Emlen et al., 1963 |
| Hexobarbital | 40 | Wistar rat (F) | Daily Fluctuation (–) ↑ | – | Sleeping time | Roberts et al., 1970 |
| | 125 | NIH mouse (M) | | – | Sleeping time | Vesell, 1968 |

Table 2 (Cont.)

| Drugs | Doses (mg/kg) (i.p.) | Species and Sex | Types of Administration When Maximum Response was Shown to Drug | | Ratio of Crest to Trough | Variables Investigated | References |
|---|---|---|---|---|---|---|---|
| | | | Light Period | Dark Period | | | |
| | 125 | Swiss–Webster mouse (M) | ← | | — | Duration of sleep | Holcslaw et al., 1975 |
| | 150 | Wistar rat (M) | | ← | — | Sleeping time | Müller, 1971, 1974 Nair and Casper, 1969; Nair, 1974 |
| | 150 | S.D. rat (M) | ← | | — | Duration of sleep | |
| Phenobarbital | 190 | Wistar rat (M) | ← | | — | Sleeping time | Müller, 1971, 1974 |
| Ethanol | 2 | NMRI mouse (M) | *Crest 12:00 (light 6:00–22:00) | | — | Sliding angle of tilted plane | Lagerspetz, 1972 |
| P-chlormeth-amphetamine | 0.5 | S.D. rat (M) | ← | | — | Avoidance response | Evans et al., 1973 |
| | 4.0 | S.D. rat (M) | ← | | — | Avoidance response | |
| Methamphetamine | 0.2 | S.D. rat (M) | | ← | — | Avoidance response | Evans et al., 1973 |
| | 1.6 | S.D. rat (M) | | ← | — | Avoidance response | |
| D-amphetamine | 1.5 | S.D. rat (M) | ← | | — | Locomotor activity | Wolfe et al., 1977 |
| | 5.0 | Wistar rat (infant) | *Crest 22:00–2:00 (light 8:00–17:00) | | — | Head-shaking | Urba–Holmgren et al., 1977 |

| Agent | Dose | Species | | Value | Effect | Reference |
|---|---|---|---|---|---|---|
| Tetrabenazine | 50.0 | S.D. rat (M) | ↑ | 2.0 | Duration of sedation | Nagayama et al., 1974, 1977 |
| Chlorpromazine | 2.5 | S.D. rat (M) | ↑ | 3.1 | Sedation period | Nagayama et al., 1977, 1978c |
| | 5.0 | S.D. rat (M) | ↑ | 2.9 | Sedation period | |
| | 10.0 | S.D. rat (M) | ↑ | 2.1 | Sedation period | |
| | 20.0 | S.D. rat (M) | ↑ | – | Sedation period | |
| | 7.5 | S.D. rat (M) | ↑ | – | Decrease in body temperature | Wolfe et al., 1977 |
| Haloperidol | 0.12 | S.D. rat (M) | ↑ | 2.8 | Anti-apomorphine effect | Nagayama et al., 1978a |
| | 0.25 | S.D. rat (M) | ↑ | 2.0 | Anti-apomorphine effect | |
| | 0.5 | S.D. rat (M) | ↑ | 1.9 | Anti-apomorphine effect | |
| | 0.5 | S.D. rat (M) | ↑ | 1.7 | Sedation period | |
| | 1.0 | S.D. rat (M) | ↑ | 1.7 | Sedation period | |
| | 2.0 | S.D. rat (M) | ↑ | 1.8 | Sedation period | |
| | 4.0 | S.D. rat (M) | ↑ | 1.6 | Sedation period | |
| | 8.0 | S.D. rat (M) | ↑ | 1.3 | Sedation period | |

* All agents, except asterisked ones, were used in an experiment with a 12-hour light and a 12-hour dark period in a day. In this table, all the times are expressed as relative clock times counted from the beginning of the light.

Comparison was made between the fluctuation of this effect and of the lethality rate. For example, pentobarbital was compared between Tables 1 and 2. Almost all the data on the lethality rate formed a crest in the dark period, but those on effect did so in the light period. It is clear that the fluctuation curve of the lethality rate was different from that of effect. By the way, the notion that death may not be merely an extension of the mechanism causing sleep is in agreement with the conclusion drawn by Kalser et al. (1969) regarding hexobarbital, which was obtained from the study not related to time.

Various studies have also been made on the circadian fluctuation of effects of those drugs from inside and outside the living organism.

## 1.  Influence of Factors from Outside the Living Organisms, or Between Living Organisms

When the light-dark rhythm of the environment was modified to maintain a light period for a long time, the circadian fluctuation disappeared in the effect (duration of sleep) of pentobarbital (Davis, 1962; Scheving et al., 1968a) and hexobarbital (Holcslaw et al., 1975). Circadian fluctuation in the effect of pentobarbital also disappeared from blinded animals (Scheving et al., 1968b). It is obvious that the light-dark rhythm of the environment exerted a decisive influence upon the circadian fluctuation of the effect of a drug.

In the experiment of Scheving et al. (1968b), however, an irregular fluctuation appeared both in animals held constantly in the light and in blinded animals after the disappearance of the circadian fluctuation. This result was probably due to some group synchronization that might have occurred in the rhythm, which had originally shown a free run, as mentioned by Scheving et al. In the experiment of Holcslaw et al. (1975), the reverse convention of light-dark rhythm made the fluctuation of effect disappear. This result may signify that a 14-day period of adaptation used for that experiment was too short for the reconstruction under the new condition of light and dark periods of a new curve of fluctuation in effect. Generally, there was an increase in reactivity in blinded animals, as well as in animals kept constantly in the light. The reason for the increase is unknown.

As an environmental condition other than light and dark, room temperature was examined. At a high temperature (36 C), a considerable leveling off of the pattern was presented. When isolated animals at the time of experiment were compared with those in groups, a circadian fluctuation of effect was exhibited by both groups of animals. When pentobarbital was administered, it was elucidated that the crest was significantly larger in value in the grouped animals than in the isolated ones (Davis, 1962).

## 2.  Influence of Factors from Inside the Living Organism

Many investigators have agreed to the opinion that there is a circadian rhythm in the drug-metabolizing activity of the liver with hexobarbital (Radzialowski et al., 1968; Vesell, 1968; Nair and Casper, 1969; Roberts et al., 1970; Jori et al., 1971; Müller, 1971, 1974; Holcslaw et al., 1975). They are also in agreement, to a considerable extent, as to the wave pattern of this rhythm. On the basis of the lengths of the light and dark periods and the number of measurements performed, comparison could be made among the experiments conducted by five of the groups of investigators cited above. The five groups of investigators agreed in finding a trough during the light period (Vesell, 1968; Nair and Casper, 1969; Jori et al., 1971; Müller, 1974), or in the transitional stage from the light to the dark period (Roberts et al., 1970).

When the light and the dark periods were reversed for a long time, the metabolic rhythm was reversed accordingly (Jori et al., 1971; Holcslaw et al., 1975). This rhythm disappeared under a constant light or dark condition (Nair and Casper, 1969; Holcslaw et al., 1975). In short, it had the same characteristics as the rhythm of duration of sleep when barbiturates were administered. The wave pattern of this rhythm is the reverse of that of the rhythm of duration of sleep with the same drug (Vesell, 1968; Nair and Casper, 1969; Müller, 1974; Holcslaw et al., 1975). That rhythm is related to changes in the ultrastructure of the liver (Nair, 1974). It is maintained, but shows a phase shift in animals subjected to bilateral superior cervical ganglionectomy, or regulated hourly feeding. It disappears in animals with medial or lateral hypothalamic lesions. Therefore, it has been reported that the rhythm is regulated by the hypothalamic centers and is partially dependent on the sympathetic innervation to the pineal gland (Nair et al., 1970).

In addition to hexobarbital, imipramine also gave rise to a circadian rhythm of metabolism. A trough appeared at the beginning of the light period, or at $3\frac{1}{2}$ hours of illumination. When the light and dark periods were reversed, this rhythm was also reversed (Jori et al., 1971).

From the aforementioned, it is considered that so far as hexobarbital is concerned, the rhythm of metabolism in the liver may be a cause of the circadian fluctuation of pharmacological effect. The situation, however, is actually more complicated.

Studies have been carried out to develop another rather direct method to search for a cause of the circadian fluctuation of pharmacological effectiveness. The aim of such a method is to clarify the relationship between the blood level or intracerebral concentration of a drug and the rhythm of duration of sleep after administration of the drug.

Roberts et al., (1970) found in their experiment that the crest of the circadian rhythm of the rate of oxidation of hexobarbital agreed with the trough of the rhythm of an unmetabolized drug concentration in the brain. In their experiment, however, there was no fluctuation in the duration of sleep. From the results of their experiment, Roberts and his co-workers presumed the presence of a rhythm of susceptibility of the brain to a drug with a crest at the time mentioned above. In conjunction with Table 2, however, it is puzzling that only in their experiment was no circadian fluctuation seen in the duration of sleep.

Nelson and Halberg (1973a) selected two time points between which there was a significant difference in the duration of pentobarbital-induced sleep. They determined chronologically the serum level and the brain concentration of pentobarbital at these time points. They found no significant difference based on TODA in the serum level or the brain concentration of the drug during the time of drug-induced sleeping. There was, however, a significant difference in the serum level and the brain concentration of the drug at the time of awakening; both the level and the concentration of the drug were higher in animals showing shorter sleep than in those showing longer sleep. No definite conclusions were drawn from these results by Nelson and Halberg (1973a).

Holcslaw et al. (1975) pointed out that when the duration of hexobarbital-induced sleep was short, the metabolic rate of this drug was rather high, as well as the intracerebral concentration of the same drug at the time of awakening. From these results, Holcslaw and his co-workers suggest that the drug susceptibility of the central nervous system and the rhythm of metabolism in the liver might be related to the circadian fluctuation of duration of sleep.

All the data mentioned above can be summarized in the following manner when the interpretation of data by the respective authors is disregarded. Namely, after administration of hexobarbital or pentobarbital, the metabolic rate was high when the duration of sleep was short, but there was no difference according to TODA in chronological changes in the blood level, or intracerebral concentration of the drug during the period of sleeping. These results can be explained as follows: There is a difference in the rate of metabolism in the liver according to TODA. However, this difference seems to have been compensated by the intervention of some other mechanism, and failed to be reflected in the blood level or intracerebral concentration of the drug. A rhythm of absorption and excretion could be considered as an example of such a mechanism. For example, a diurnal fluctuation was found in the excretion of methylamphetamine (Beckett et al., 1964). Since the concentration of a drug distributed in the brain was the same, regardless of TODA, it is reasonable to assume that the difference in the duration of sleep between any two TODA's may have been induced by the circadian rhythm in the drug susceptibility of the brain. This assumption is also supported by the results that there was a difference based on TODA in the intracerebral concentration of the drug at the time of awakening, and that this concentration was significantly high when the duration of sleep was short.

## D. CIRCADIAN FLUCTUATION IN EFFECTS OF NEUROLEPTICS INDUCED BY DIFFERENCE IN TODA

As shown in Table 2, with a single exception (Wolfe et al., 1977), all the experiments mentioned in this section were carried out at the author's laboratory. The three drugs used—tetrabenazine, chlorpromazine, and haloperidol—were different in action mechanism. Another experiment was conducted with apomorphine, since it was also closely related. In this section, a large amount of unpublished data is cited in addition to published data (Nagayama et al., 1974, 1975, 1977a, 1977b, 1978a, 1978b; Takagi et al., 1976).

In the experiment, male rats of Sprague-Dawley (S.D.) strain weighing 300 to 400 g were used. For at least 5 weeks before the beginning of the experiment, they were raised at temperatures from 24 to 26 C and exposed to light for only 12 hours daily, or from 7:30 P.M. to 7:30 A.M. Each rat was used only once in the experiment.

### 1. Circadian Fluctuation in Sedative Effect

A rat was placed in a semi-soundproof experimental box, which was kept at the same temperature and illuminated in the same manner as in the animal room, at 4:30 P.M. The rat was allowed 27 to 48 hours to adapt itself to the box. Then it was administered a drug warmed at 24 C. The amount of locomotion was determined with the apparatus Animex (an A.B. Farard product). Accordingly, the experiment was carried out under strictly controlled conditions, where the rat was protected from any disturbance by external stimulation from the beginning to the end of the experiment, except at the time of drug administration. As an indicator of sedative effect, the sedation period, or the duration of sedation caused by the drug, was measured. In this measurement, a perfectly objective indicator was set up to allow no room for any subjective evaluation to take place. The indicator was an interval of time required for the apparatus Animex to record 90 counts per 10 minutes after the appearance of sedation.

The rats were injected intraperitoneally with the drug at varying times. As a result, a significant circadian fluctuation in sedative effect was noticed after injection with tetrabenazine (Nagayama et al., 1974, 1977b), chlorpromazine (Nagayama et al., 1977a, 1978c), and haloperidol (Nagayama et al., 1978a).

This experiment was characteristic, since a great many doses of the same drug were used extensively, and a circadian fluctuation in effect was determined for every dose. For example, chlorpromazine gave rise to a dose-response curve, as shown in Figure 1. In this figure, the pattern of fluctuation varies with the dose of the drug. When a small dose was injected, susceptibility was the highest at 1:30 A.M. (TODA) and decreased in the order listed at 7:30 P.M. 1:30 P.M., and 7:30 A.M.. When a large dose was injected, the maximum response was the most outstanding at 7:30 A.M. and decreased in the order listed at 1:30 P.M., 7:30 P.M., and 1:30 A.M., showing a circadian fluctuation.

Figure 2 is the schematic presentation of these results. It indicates that the curve of susceptibility is the mirror image of the curve of the maximum response. In brief, the wave pattern of the curve of circadian fluctuation varied with the dose of the drug. This phenomenon was also observed when haloperidol was administered. Table 2 shows the realtionship between the dose of haloperidol administered and the appearance of a crest in the curve of fluctuation.

On the other hand, a circadian fluctuation was also noticed in the lethality rate of chlorpromazine. In this case, a crest appeared at 7:30 P.M.. It was compared with the crest of the curve of sedative effect. Figure 3 presents a curve of fluctuation for each dose of administration drawn on the basis of

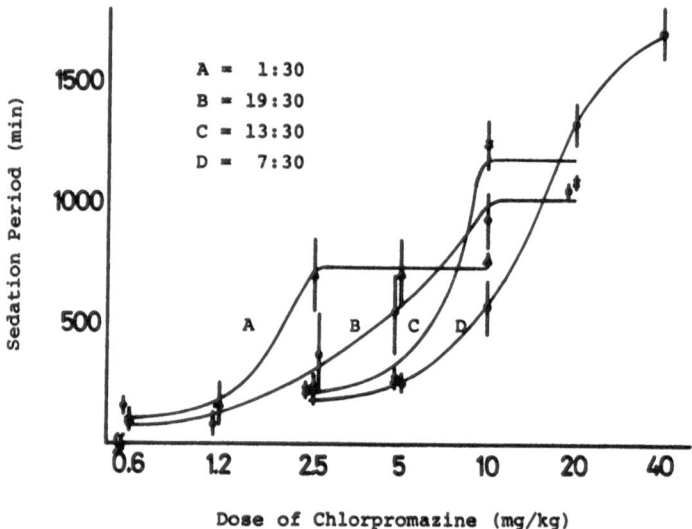

**Figure 1.** Dose-response curves by time of chlorpromazine administration. Each point represents mean ± SE. Significant differences are found between each curve. Analysis of variance: $p < 0.005$.

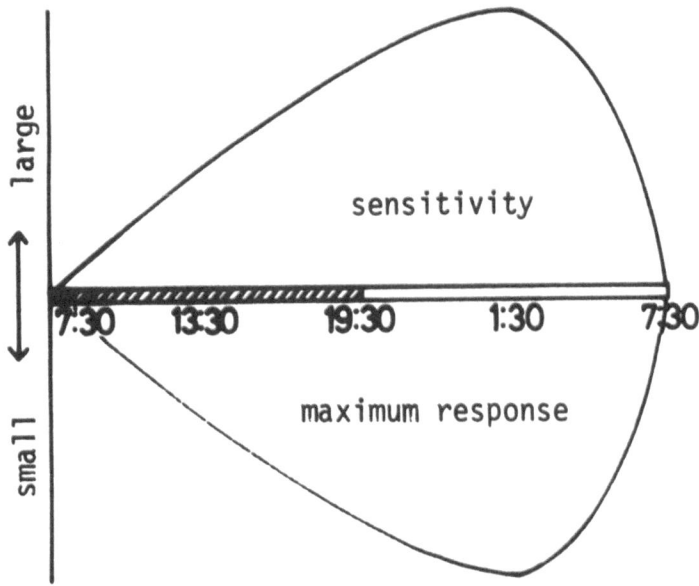

**Figure 2.** Schematic presentation of daily fluctuation of sensitivity and maximum response to chlorpromazine.

data given in Figure 1. The crest of sedative effect moved gradually and smoothly, in accordance with an increase in dose of administration, from 1:30 A.M. (2.5 mg/kg) to 7:30 P.M., and from 1:30 P.M. to 7:30 A.M. (20 mg/kg), or from the middle of the light period to the end of the dark period and further to the beginning of the dark period. On the other hand, the crest of the lethality rate (74 mg/kg) was not on the line extended in the moving direction of that crest. Therefore, the circadian fluctuation of effect seems to be a phenomenon different from that of lethality rate and appears to be under rules different from those for the latter (Nagayama et al., 1978c).

To search for external factors controlling the circadian fluctuation of effect, the rats were exposed to the reversed light and dark periods throughout the preliminary and the proper experimental periods. During these reversals, the curve of circadian fluctuation of sedative effect was also completely reversed. Therefore, it was made clear that the circadian fluctuation of effect was controlled externally by the light-dark rhythm. On the other hand, it was noticed that there were two time points, between which a significant difference in effect of the drug was observed during the same dark period. Accordingly, it was elucidated that animals did not respond simply to light or dark, but exhibited a response to the relative hour produced by the light-dark rhythm (Nagayama et al., 1978c).

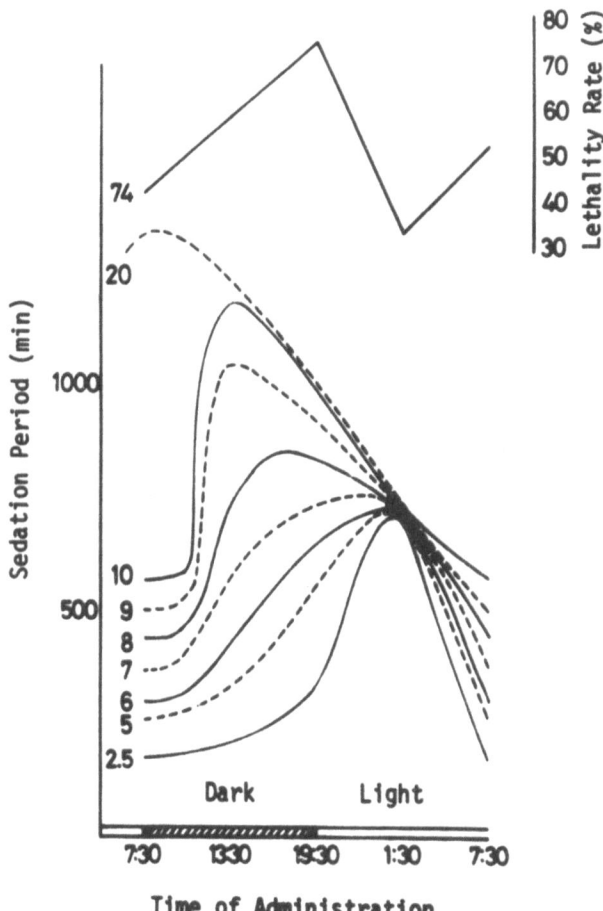

**Figure 3.** Daily fluctuation of sedation period by chlorpromazine dose and lethality rate. Figures at the left end of each curve denote doses of chlorpromazine. Sedation period at each dose from 2.5–20 mg/kg and lethality rate at 74 mg/kg.

## 2.  Chronological Changes of Blood Level and Intracerebral Concentration of Drug and Circadian Fluctuation of Sedative Effect

An experiment was carried out to clarify the mechanism of appearance of a circadian fluctuation of sedative effect of a drug. In it, two time points that had a significant difference in the sedative effect of the drug were selected. The blood level and intracerebral concentration of the drug were measured at regular intervals after administration of the drug. Tetrabenazine (Nagayama et al., 1974, 1977b), chlorpromazine (Nagayama et al., 1977a, 1978c), and haloperidol (Nagayama et al., 1978a) were administered;

there was no difference in the rise and fall of blood level of intracerebral concentration based on TODA. The same determination was also reached with demethylated chlorpromazine and chlorpromazine sulfoxide, which are principal metabolites of chlorpromazine; there was no difference based on TODA either in the blood level or intracerebral concentration. These results indicate that the circadian fluctuation of sedative effect of these drugs is not dependent upon the circadian fluctuation of level of absorption, excretion, metabolism, or distribution of the drugs. Nevertheless, it is of course possible that there may be a circadian fluctuation in the levels of absorption, excretion, and metabolism of the drugs, which is being counteracted by a mutual antagonism of these rhythms or by the intervention of some other mechanism, thereby maintaining a constant blood level of the drug. At any rate, it is true that the same concentration of the drug is distributed in the brain, regardless of TODA. This fact seems to indicate that the circadian fluctuation of sedative effect of the drug was not induced by these peripheral mechanisms, but by the circadian rhythm of drug sensitivity of the brain, at the site of action of the drug.

It is also possible to surmise that the cause of this circadian fluctuation of sedative effect of the drug may emerge at the time when such non-specific stimulation as injection was given without connection to the drug itself. This hypothesis, however, is negated by the fact that the pattern of fluctuation varies with the kind of drug and, as shown in Figure 3, with the dose of administration.

To elucidate the mechanism that induces the rhythm of drug sensitivity more distinctly, it is necessary to study the intracerebral action mechanism of the drug. Further discussion centers chiefly on haloperidol.

It has been reported that haloperidol displays its action by blocking dopamine receptors, as well as norepinephrine receptors, in the brain. Its principal action is presumed to be derived from blocking dopamine receptors (Andén et al., 1970). To clarify the relationship between the action of haloperidol and dopamine receptors, some issues must be resolved. They are concerned with the presence or absence of a circadian rhythm in the amount of dopamine contained in the brain; the presence or absence of a circadian rhythm in the sensitivity of dopamine receptors to dopamine; and finally, the presence or absence of a circadian fluctuation in the action of haloperidol to block dopamine receptors. It has already been shown that there is no circadian rhythm in the amount of dopamine contained in the brain (Scheving et al., 1968a; Simon and George, 1975). So we can move on to the question of the presence or absence of a circadian rhythm in the sensitivity of the dopamine receptors to dopamine.

### 3. Circadian Fluctuation of Effect of Apomorphine

To examine the sensitivity of dopamine receptors in the brain, apomorphine was administered at varying times, and response to it was determined with the duration of apomorphine-induced stereotyped behavior (AISB) as an indicator. Apomorphine has been reported to be an agonist of dopamine and to stimulate the receptors of this amine directly (Andén et al., 1967; Ernst, 1967; Kehr et al., 1972; Lahti et al., 1972; Nybäck et al., 1970; Roos, 1969). With doses of 0.6 to 80.0 mg/kg of apomorphine, the duration of AISB showed a circadian fluctuation with a crest and a trough appearing at 7:30 P.M. and 1:30 P.M., respectively. Then, an attempt was made to determine whether this circadian fluctuation was brought about by a difference in sensitivity of receptors, or in concentration of apomorphine in the brain. The drug was administered at two time points between which there was a significant difference in the duration of AISB, and the intracerebral concentration of the drug was measured at regular intervals at given different sites of the brain such as the cortex, the striatum, the hypothalamus, mid-brain, and the pons. No difference in concentration was seen between such time points at any site, which was directly related to the action of the drug. In short, the same concentration of apomorphine was present at the sites of action in the brain, regardless of TODA. It was thus clarified that the circadian fluctuation of AISB was caused by that of sensitivity to the drug at the site of action (Nagayama et al., 1978b). In conclusion, the sensitivity of dopamine receptors in the brain presented a circadian rhythm with a crest and a trough at 7:30 P.M. and 1:30 P.M., respectively. The question remains: What happens when neuroleptics act upon these receptors?

## 4.   Circadian Fluctuation in Action of Drug to Block Dopamine Receptors in the Brain

AISB was determined in animals administered with 5 mg/kg of apomorphine 1 hour after administration of haloperidol. It was also determined in other animals after administration of a combination of apomorphine and physiological saline. In this manner, it was possible to calculate a rate at which AISB was inhibited by haloperidol. As a result, this rate was found to have a circadian fluctuation with a crest at 7:30 P.M. and a trough at 1:30 P.M.. There was no relationship between this pattern of fluctuation and the dose (0.12 to 0.5 mg/kg) of haloperidol used (Nagayama et al., 1978a).

Next, comparison was made between the curve of fluctuation of sedative effect of haloperidol and that of the rate of AISB inhibition. Since this rate was estimated with a small dose of haloperidol, it was necessary to use the curve of fluctuation of sedative effect for an equally small dose for comparison. As a result, both curves of fluctuation were almost identical (Figure 4). They presented essentially the same pattern that showed a crest at

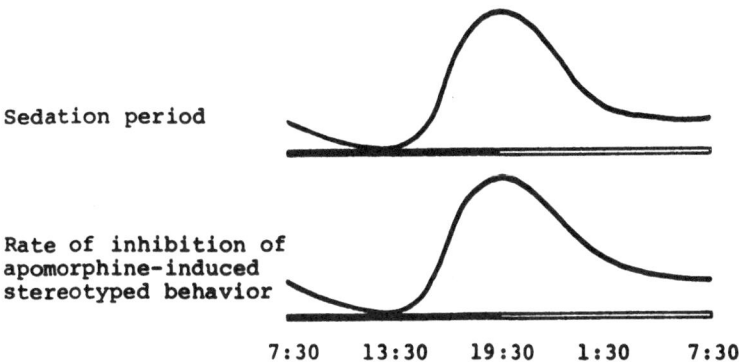

Sedation period

Rate of inhibition of
apomorphine-induced
stereotyped behavior

7:30      13:30      19:30      1:30      7:30

**Figure 4.** Comparison of daily fluctuations in sedative effect and anti-apomorphine effect of haloperidol (0.5 mg/kg).

first at 7:30 P.M. and then a decline in the order listed at 1:30 A.M., 7:30 A.M., and 1:30 P.M.. This pattern can hardly be regarded as an incidental one, and seems to suggest that in the case of haloperidol, a circadian fluctuation in the sedative effect was induced by the circadian fluctuation in the rate of blocking dopamine receptors in the brain by haloperidol.

Why did the pattern of circadian fluctuation in sedative effect vary with the dose of the drug administered? In the above-mentioned dose-response curve of the sedative effect of haloperidol, the circadian fluctuation in the case of administration of a small dose of the drug is assumed to have been induced by the circadian rhythm of affinity of dopamine receptors in the brain. In addition, the circadian fluctuation in the maximum response in the case of administration of a large dose of the drug is assumed to have been induced by the circadian fluctuation in the number of binding sites of these receptors. It seems that the rate of AISB inhibition by chlorpromazine may present a different curve of fluctuation (Nagayama et al., 1978a). It is presumed that the circadian fluctuation of sedative effect of tetrabenazine may be explained (Nagayama et al., 1977b) by the fact that the sedative action of this drug is caused by an increase in serotonin in synapses (Tachiki et al., 1978), and by an assumption that a diurnal fluctuation may occur in the capacity of releasing serotonin (Héry et al., 1972). Even for phenomena such as the circadian fluctuation of sedative effect, the mechanism of appearance may vary with the kind of drug in relation to the action mechanism of the respective drug. Incidentally, Wolfe et al. (1977) found that there was circadian fluctuation in the chlorpromazine-induced hypothermia, and that measurement of in vivo disposition (brain and plasma) of the drug did not vary at different times of day. These authors reported that the temporal variations observed in response to chlorpromazine do not result from alterations in drug disposition, but may reflect time-dependent changes in sensitivity of tissue to this central-nervous-system agent. Their explanation is fundamentally similar to our theory.

## E.  COMMENTS

What has been clarified so far about the circadian fluctuation in the effects of neuroleptics is summarized as follows. Indeed, such clarified fluctuation has been confirmed only in three drugs up to this time, but it is believed that this fluctuation will be observed rather extensively in drugs at large, since the three drugs were selected as representatives from groups of drugs each exhibiting a different action mechanism.

1. There was circadian fluctuation in the effects of neuroleptics.
2. The curve of circadian fluctuation of the effect of a drug varied in wave pattern with the kind of drug used.
3. The curve of circadian fluctuation of the effect of a drug varied in wave pattern with the size of the dose.
4. A circadian fluctuation was found in lethality rate. It formed a curve different from the one for the circadian fluctuation of the effect of a drug and seemed to be controlled by a law different from that controlling this fluctuation.
5. The circadian fluctuation of the effect of a drug was regulated externally by the relative hour produced by the light-dark rhythm.
6. The circadian fluctuation of the effect of a drug was regulated internally, not by the concentration of the drug in the brain, but by the circadian rhythm of sensitivity of the brain to the drug.

The present studies on such phenomena as the circadian fluctuation of the effects of neuroleptics are of great significance. First, they point out the importance of the time of drug administration in many experiments where a drug must be administered to living organisms. As shown in Tables 1 and 2, there are differences amounting to several times the effect and toxicity of a drug between any two time points of administration. This finding casts doubt upon the results of an experiment where the importance of TODA was disregarded. In this connection, since the "time" in this sense is formed by a regular light and dark rhythm, a strict control on this rhythm becomes a basic, indispensable condition for animal experiments.

Secondly, such phenomena as the circadian fluctuation of the effect of a drug may serve as a useful means for the clarification of the action mechanism of neuroleptics. It is necessary to use various neuroleptics to elucidate common points, as well as different points, in the circadian fluctuation of the physiological and biochemical effects of these drugs, as well as the fluctuation of the effects from the standpoint of behavioral science.

Thirdly, such studies will be a useful means for studying the essential nature of a biological clock, if one does exist.

Lastly, from the standpoint of clinical usefulness, if a curve of circadian fluctuation can be drawn for the effect of each drug, it will be possible to adjust the dose of administration for a given time of administration by referring to the curve. Then it will be possible to carry out a more effective treatment than the conventional one, which is generally performed without any definite basis, by dividing the daily dose of a drug into three equal portions to medicate three times a day. On the other hand, attempts have recently been made in many areas to administer single daily doses of neuroleptics (Dimascio and Shader, 1969); and here too, the circadian fluctuation of the effect of a drug may be applicable. Until now, it has been used mainly to decrease the time required for drug administration and to reduce the bother of drug administration for the patient. Therefore, many conventional studies have been conducted mostly to disprove any negative points of treatment, such as exacerbated symptoms or increase in side effects. Nevertheless, a positive approach may be made in search of the effects of many drugs by utilizing the circadina fluctuation of the effect of a drug. Of the many effects of a drug, some may present an individual pattern of fluctuation. Therefore, it seems necessary to determine a TODA when as many effects and as few side effects of the drug as possible are expected. As mentioned above, at least sedative effect and lethality rate presented different patterns of fluctuation. Judging from this result, it seems quite certain that a diurnal fluctuation may exist in a margin of safety ($LD_{50}/ED_{50}$).

Such phenomena as the circadian fluctuation of pharmacological effect is no longer considered as wondrous. The time has come to clarify the laws controlling this phenomenon and to study its practical implication for treatment.

## F. REFERENCES

Andén, N.-E., Butcher, S.G., Corrodi, H., Fuxe, K., and Ungerstedt, U. (1970). Receptor activity and turnover of dopamine and noradrenaline after neuroleptics. *Eur. J. Pharmacol.* 11:303-314.

Andén, N.-E., Rubenson, A., Fuxe, K. and Hökfelt, T. (1967). Evidence for dopamine receptor stimulation by apomorphine. *J. Pharm. Pharmacol.* 19:627-629.

Beckett, A.H., and Rowland, M. (1964). Rhythmic urinary excretion of amphetamine in man. *Nat.* 204:1203-1204.

Davies, J.A., and Redfern, P.H. (1973). The effect of hallucinogenic drugs on maze exploration in the rat over a 24-hour period. *Brit. J. Pharmacol.* 49:121-127.

Davis, W.M. (1962). Day-night periodicity in pentobarbital response of mice and the influence of socio-psychological conditions. *Experientia.* 18:235-237.

Dimascio, A., and Shader, R.I. (1969). Drug administration schedules. *Am. J. Psychiat.* 126:796-801.

Emlen, S.T., and Kem, W. (1963). Activity rhythm in peromyscus: Its influence on rats of recovery from nembutal. *Sci.* 142:1682-1683.

Ernst, A.M. (1967). Mode of action of apomorphine and dexamphetamine on gnawing compulsion in rats. *Psychopharmacologia.* 10:316-323.

Evans, H.L., Ghiselli, W.B., and Patton, R.A. (1973). Diurnal rhythm in behavioral effects of methamphetamine, P-chloromethamphetamine, and scopolamine. *J. Pharmacol. Exper. Therapeut.* 186:10-17.

Friedman, A.H., and Walker, C.A. (1969). Rat brain amines, blood histamine, and glucose levels in relationship to circadian changes in sleep induced by pentobarbitone sodium. *J. Physiol.* 202:133-146.

Hata, T., Okage, T., Miyake, Y., and Kita, T. (1975). Relationship between administration time of drugs and acute toxicity in mice. *Fol. Pharmacolog. Jap.* 71:29-37.

Haus, E., and Halberg, F. (1959). 24-hour rhythm in susceptibility of C mice to a toxic dose of ethanol. *J. App. Physiol.* 14:878-880.

Hawkins, R., Kripke, D.F., and Janowsky, D.S. (1978). Circadian rhythm of lithium toxicity in mice. *Psychopharmacol.* 56:113-114.

Héry, F., Rouer, E., and Glowinski, J. (1972). Daily variations of serotonin metabolism in the rat brain. *Brain Res.* 43:445-465.

Holcslaw, T.L., Miya, T.S., and Bousquet, W.S. (1975). Circadian rhythms in drug action and drug metabolism in the mouse. *J. Pharmacol. Exper. Therapeut.* 195:320-332.

Jori, A., Di Salle, E., and Santini, V. (1971). Daily rhythmic variation and liver drug metabolism in rats. *Biochem. Pharmacol.* 20:2965-2969.

Kalser, S.C., Forbes, E., and Kunig, R. (1969). Relation of brain sensitivity and hepatic metabolism of hexobarbitone to dose-response relations in infant and young rats. *J. Pharm. Pharmacol.* 21:109-113.

Kehr, W., Carlsson, A., Lindqvist, M., Magnusson, J., and Atack, C. (1972). Evidence for a receptor-mediated feedback control of striatal tyrosine hydroxylase activity. *J. Pharm. Pharmacol.* 24:744-747.

Lagerspetz, K.Y.H. (1972). Diurnal variation in the effect of alcohol and in the brain 5-hydroxytryptamine metabolism in mice. *Acta Pharmacolog. Toxicolog.* 31:509-520.

Lahti, R.A., McAllister, B., and Wozniak, J. (1972). Apomorphine antagonist of the elevation of homovanillic acid induced by antipsychotic drugs. *Life Sci.* 11:605-613.

Lindsay, H.A., and Kullman, V.S. (1966). Pentobarbital sodium. Variation in toxicity. *Sci.* 151:576-577.

Marte, E., and Halberg, F. (1961). Circadian susceptibility rhythm of mice to librium. *Fed. Proc.* 20:305.

Moore Ede, M.C. (1973). Circadian rhythm of drug effectiveness and toxicity. *Clin. Pharmacol. Therapeut.* 14:925-935.

Müller, O. (1974). Circadian rhythmicity in response to barbiturates, in *Chronobiology.* L.E. Scheving, F. Halberg, and J.E. Pauly, eds. Igaku Shoin, Tokyo. pp. 187-190.

Müller, O. (1971). Circadian rhythmicity in response to barbiturates. *Naunyn-Schmiedeberg's Arch. Pharmacol.* 270: Supp. R 99.

Nagayama, H., Takagi, A., and Takahashi, R. (1978a). (Unpublished data).

Nagayama, H., Takagi, A., Nakamura, E., Yoshida, H., and Takahashi, R. (1978b). (submitted for publication). Circadian susceptibility rhythm to apomorphine in the brain. *Comm. Psychopharmacol.*

Nagayama, H., Takagi, A., Nishiwaki, K., and Takahashi, R. (1977a). Studies on the susceptibility rhythm in rat to chlorpromazine. *Ann. Rep. Pharmacopsychiat. Res. Found.* 8:267-271.

Nagayama, H., Takagi, A., Sakurai, Y., Nishiwaki, K., and Takahashi, R. (1978c). Chronopharmacological study of neuroleptics. II. Circadian susceptibility rhythm to chlorproma-zine. *Psychopharmacol.* 58:49-53.

Nagayama, H., Takagi, A., Tateishi, T., and Takahashi, R. (1977b). Circadian susceptibility rhythm to neuroleptics: Tetrabenazine. *Psychopharmacol.* 55:61-66.

Nagayama, H., Takagi, A., Tateishi, T., and Takahashi, R. (1975). Studies on the situational factors affecting the effect of psychotropic drugs. I. Daily fluctuation of sedative effect of tetrabenazine. *Psychiat. Neurolog. Jap.* 77:925-932.

Nagayama, H., Takagi, A., Tateishi, T., and Takahashi, R. (1974). Studies on diurnal fluctuation of sedative effect of tetrabenazine. *Jap. J. Pharmacol.* 24:112.

Nair, V. (1974). Circadian rhythm in drug action; a pharmacologic, biochemical, and electro-microscopic study, in *Chronobiology.* L.E. Scheving, F. Halberg, and J.E. Pauly, eds. Igaku Shoin, Tokyo. pp. 182-186.

Nair, V., and Casper, R. (1969). The influence of light on daily rhythm in hepatic drug metabolizing enzymes in rats. *Life Sci.* 8:1291-1298.

Nair, V., Casper, R., Siegel, S., and Bau, D. (1970). Regulation of the diurnal rhythm in hepatic drug metabolism. *Fed. Proc.* 29:804.

Nelson, W., and Halberg, F. (1973a). An evaluation of time-dependent changes in susceptibility of mice to pentobarbital injection. *Neuropharmacol.* 12:509-524.

Nelson, W., and Halberg, F. (1973b). Effects of a synchronizer phase-shift on circadian rhythms in response of mice to ethanol or ouabain. *Space Life Sci.* 4:249-257.

Nybäck, H., Schubert, J., and Sedvall, G. (1970). Effect of apomorphine and pimozide on synthesis and turnover of labelled catecholamines in mouse brain. *J. Pharm. Pharmacol.* 22:622-624.

Pauly, J., and Scheving, L.E. (1964). Temporal variations in the susceptibility of white rats to pentobarbital sodium and tremorine. *Int. J. Neuropharmacol.* 3:651-658.

Radzialowski, F., and Bousquet, W. (1968). Daily rhythmic variation in hepatic drug metabo-lism in the rat and mouse. *J. Pharmacol. Exper. Therapeut.* 163:229-238.

Reinberg, A. (1973). Chronopharmacology, in *Biochemical Aspects of Circadian Rhythms.* J.N. Mills, ed. Plenum Press, London. pp. 121 152.

Roberts, P., Turnbull, M.J., and Winterburn, A. (1970). Diurnal variation in sensitivity to and metabolism of barbiturate in the rat: Lack of correlation between in vivo and in vitro findings. *Eur. J. Pharmacol.* 12:375-377.

Roos, B.-E. (1969). Decrease in homovanillic acid as evidence for dopamine receptor stimula-tion by apomorphine in the neostriatum of the rat. *J. Pharm. Pharmacol.* 21:263-264.

Scheving, L.E. (1969). Circadian variation in susceptibility of the rat to d-amphetamine sulfate. *Anatom. Rec.* 160:422.

Scheving, L.E. (1968). Daily circadian rhythm in rats to d-amphetamine sulphate. Effect of blinding and continuous illumination on the rhythm. *Nat.* 219:621-622.

Scheving, L.E., Harrison, W.H., Gordon, P., and Pauly, J.E. (1968a). Daily fluctuation (circadian and ultradian) in biogenic amines of the rat brain. *Am. J. Physiol.* 214:166-173.

Scheving, L.E., Vedral, D.F., and Pauly, J.E. (1968b). A circadian susceptibility rhythm in rats to pentobarbital sodium. *Anatom. Rec.* 160:741-749.

Simon, M.L., and George, R. (1975). Diurnal variations in plasma corticosterone and growth hormone as correlated with regional variations in norepinephrine, dopamine, and sero-tonin content of rat brain. *Neuroendocrinol.* 17:125-138.

Tachiki, K.H., Takagi, A., Tateishi, T., Kido, A., Nishiwaki, K., Nakamura, E., Nagayama, H., and Takahashi, R. (1978). Animal model of depression. III. Mechanism of action of tetrabenazine. *Biolog. Psychiat.* 13:429-443.

Takagi, A., Nagayama, H., Sakurai, Y., Tateishi, T., and Takahashi, R. (1976). Daily fluctuation of sedative effect of a psychotropic drug (chlorpromazine). *Ann. Rep. Phar-macopsychiat. Res. Found.* 7:168-171.

Urba-Holmgren, R., Holmgren, B., and Aquiar, M. (1977). Circadian variation in an amphetamine induced motor response. *Pharmacol. Biochem. Behav.* 7:571-572.

Vesell, E.S. (1968). Genetic and environmental factors affecting hexobarbital metabolism in mice. *Ann. N. Y. Acad. Sci.* 151:900-912.

Walker, C. (1974). Implications of biological rhythms in brain amine concentrations and drug toxicity, in *Chronobiology*. L.E. Scheving, F. Halberg, and J.E. Pauly, eds. Igaku Shoin, Tokyo. pp. 205-208.

Walker, C.A., and Owasoyo, J.O. (1974). The influence of serotonin, GABA, and L-dopa on the circadian rhythm in the toxicity of picrotoxin, pentylenetetrazol, and phenobarbital in mice. *Int. J. Chronobiol.* 2:125-130.

Wolfe, G.W., Bousquet, W.F., and Schnell, R.C. (1977). Circadian variations in response to amphetamine and chlorpromazine in the rat. *Comm. Psychopharmacol.* 1:29-37.

# Subject Index

# Author Index